Endocrine-Immune
Mechanisms in Animals
and Human Health
Implications

A COMPENDIUM OF ARTICLES BY

ALFRED J. PLECHNER, D.V.M.

ENDOCRINE-IMMUNE
MECHANISMS IN ANIMALS AND
HUMAN HEALTH IMPLICATIONS
Copyright © 2003 Alfred J. Plechner, D.V.M

Cover and Book Design by Sherry Wachter Printed in the United States on recycled paper.

This book is intended for information only. Please contact your own healthcare professional for specific recommendations and treatment. Healthcare providers interested in further information about the clinical studies should contact Dr. Plechner.

Contents

Introduction

Large numbers of pets die or become sick before their time despite the best efforts of veterinarians. I believe much of this has to do with hormonal imbalances that destabilize and weaken animals' immune systems, undermine their natural protection against illness, and rob them of health and longevity.

Many "end-of-the-line animals" are referred to me in my clinical practice. Their owners have been told that euthanasia is the only option left. In some very advanced cases this may be true, but in a vast majority of situations there is hope because there is a solution.

Many years ago as a young practitioner I tried to figure out why so many of my patients were getting sick and not responding to standard treatments. My clinical work led me to a major hormonal-immune system disturbance that begins in the adrenal glands and goes on to create a ripple effect throughout the body's physiology, opening the door to conditions ranging from common skin allergies to reproductive failure to catastrophic autoimmune disease to cancer. By identifying and correcting this problem I created a successful program that has helped thousands of my own patients as well as many animals treated at other veterinary clinics.

The endocrine-immune imbalances I see result from an unsuspected deficiency, defect, or binding of cortisol. Whether from genetics, toxicity, stress, or combinations thereof, many animals lack active cortisol. I correct this deficiency by using very low dosages of cortisone—the pharmaceutical equivalent of the body's naturally occurring cortisol—on a long-term basis. In my practice I use both synthetic cortisone medications and a natural cortisol preparation derived from an ultra extract of soy. When used at very low dosages (often in conjunction with thyroid supplementation) they represent safe and significant healing agents for many seemingly unrelated diseases.

The protocol has been extremely effective when followed as directed on a long-term basis by pet owners. As a clinician, my patients are my primary concern. For that reason I have not conducted controlled studies where one group of patients receives treatment and another group, for comparison, receives a placebo. I cannot in good conscience deny treatment to suffering animals who I know will benefit from that treatment. Perhaps such an experiment can be done by researchers who have the means and interest.

TREATMENT PLAN FOR HUMANS

William Jefferies, M.D., emeritus clinical professor of internal medicine at the University of Virginia, pioneered long-term, low-dosage cortisone treatments for humans. Now in his eighties, Jefferies has reported for years that this method safely and effectively improves patients with allergies, chronic fatigue, and autoimmune disorders. Yet, just as in veterinary medicine, this effective treatment for humans has been generally ignored.

Until recently, Jefferies and I were not aware of our parallel work—one in human medicine, the other in veterinary medicine. We met for the first time in 2002 when I was invited to present my findings to physicians at a conference sponsored by the Broda O. Barnes M.D. Research Foundation in Trumbull, Connecticut.

Cortisone has a considerable stigma attached to it. But, as both Jefferies and I found independently, the problem of side effects relates largely to the use of powerful, pharmacologic dosages, and not to smaller, physiologic dosages. This is an important distinction. (See Figure 1 for a more detailed comparison between the functions, side effects, and benefits of pharmacologic and physiologic cortisone.) So, too, is the understanding that these small, physiologic dosages of natural cortisol or synthetic cortisone medications are used as a form of hormone replacement to compensate for a hormone defect.

My new book, *Pets at Risk: From Allergies to Cancer, Remedies for an Unsuspected Epidemic* (NewSage Press 2003), offers detailed instructions on how to perform the blood test I developed to identify cortisol-based endocrine-immune imbalances and how to translate the results into an individually calibrated and effective hormone replacement program.

If followed carefully, the program can significantly and rapidly improve even very sick animals. It is also an approach that I believe may offer significant insights for the treatment of human illnesses.

Some of the information contained in this syllabus has been published in medical and health journals; some is currently scheduled for publication at the time of this printing. My article, "Unrecognized Adrenal-Immune Disturbance in Pets Offers Therapeutic Insights for Multiple Human Disorders," was previously published under the title "Chaos in the Cortex," in the April 2003 issue of the *Townsend Letter for Doctors & Patients*. The article gives an overview of the endocrine-immune imbalance mechanism. The subsequent articles present specific perspectives: how pollution and toxicity can damage endocrine-immune homeostasis and the mechanism's involvement in infertility, vaccination complications, and cancer. Finally, I share clinical perspectives intended to be of practical help to clinicians.

I welcome communication from health professionals interested in exploring the role of endocrine-immune imbalances.

ALFRED J. PLECHNER, D.V.M.

Unrecognized Endocrine-Immune Defects in Multiple Diseases

An Effective Veterinary Model May Offer Therapeutic Promise for Human Illness

©Alfred J. Plechner, D.V.M.

For nearly three decades, I have treated multiple serious diseases in cats and dogs by correcting an unrecognized endocrine-immune imbalance caused by a cortisol deficiency or defect. The cortisol abnormality creates a domino effect on feedback loops involving the hypothalamus-pituitary-adrenal axis. Estrogen becomes elevated, thyroid hormone becomes bound, and B and T cells become deregulated. Diseases with this aberration as a primary etiological component range from allergies and strange behavior to severe cases of autoimmunity and cancer. I have consistently and successfully treated and controlled the condition, even in critical cases, with a long-term physiological (not pharmacological) cortisone replacement combined with thyroid hormone (in dogs). The treatment represents a major healing modality for many seemingly unrelated chronic animal diseases. In humans, this endocrine-immune dysfunction appears to exist and, as in veterinary medicine, has been overlooked by researchers and clinicians. Testing and treatment patterned after the animal model may offer significant clinical benefits for challenging human afflictions.

***

Years ago, as a new practitioner, I became frustrated by the constant battle with canine and feline allergies and diseases for which medical training provided little guidance other than treating symptoms. In an attempt to understand causality and explore the possibility of more effective treatments I began my own clinical research.

In both young and old animals, I frequently found similar problems among littermates and along familial lines: severe hypersensitivity, widespread inflamed skin, ulcerations and pruritis, malabsorption, and out of control internal systems. The path of inquiry led to the strong suspicion that contemporary breeding practices were causing narrowed gene pools, compromised health, and decreased lifespan.

For many conditions involving inflammation and pruritis, veterinary medicine commonly relies on an effective family of cortisol-type drugs (cortisone) for short-term therapy. As with human medicine, however, there is considerable reluctance about using these drugs long-term because of well-known side effects. Even with this concern in mind, I reasoned that cortisone therapy might in some way address an endocrine abnormality due to an unexplained genetic disturbance. Since cortisone is an adrenal hormone replacement, my attention turned to the adrenal glands.

Continued investigations indicated the presence of an unrecognized genetic flaw involving two of the three layers of the adrenal cortex and differing from the classic Addison's and Cushing's syndromes. Specifically, I found a problem in cortisol production causing a significant and damaging domino effect on other hormones and the immune system. Cortisol, the primary adrenal glucocorticoid, is produced in the middle cortex layer. This critical hormone stimulates several processes that serve to increase and maintain normal concentrations of glucose in blood, exerts a potent anti-inflammatory effect, and acts as a regulating factor for normal immune function.

Cortisol is secreted in response to a single stimulator: adrenocorticotropic hormone (ACTH) from the anterior pituitary. ACTH is itself secreted under control of the hypothalamic corticotropic-releasing factor (CRF). Cortisol secretion is suppressed or stimulated by classical feedback loops. When blood concentrations rise above a certain threshold, cortisol inhibits CRF secretion. This, in turn, inhibits ACTH and cortisol secretion.

However, when the adrenal gland is unable to produce enough cortisol, or for some reason the cortisol is bound and therefore not recognized by the system, the pituitary continues to produce ACTH in order to extract more cortisol.

The inner cortical layer, where adrenal estrogen is produced, also responds to ACTH. Constant ACTH stimulation in a situation where cortisol is bound or deficient produces a release of adrenal estrogen into the system. The estrogen activates a direct feedback on the hypothalamus. CRF is induced to stimulate the pituitary to release ACTH, releasing yet more estrogen from the inner layer of the adrenal cortex and raising the level of total estrogen in the system.

The influence of excess estrogen is a major confounding factor, causing the following: a histamine-like effect on capillaries, leading to inflammation from blood components spilling into adjacent tissue; binding of thyroid hormone and cortisol; and further deregulation of lymphocytes and antibodies.

I relate the loss of critical immune system function to poor resistance and immune cells which cannot properly defend against viral, bacterial, and fungal infections, or protect the body against cancer. The regulation loss is probably related to autoimmune damage, as well. Repeated clinical testing has shown that the endocrine imbalance described here coincides with abnormal levels of IgA, IgG, and IgM immunoglobulins.

The outer adrenal cortical layer, where the mineralcorticoid hormone is manufactured, appears to play no discernible role in this endocrine-immune derangement. A deficiency of mineralcorticoid secretion, which governs sodium and potassium levels, is associated with Addison's disease. An excess of cortisol is the biomarker for Cushing's syndrome.

Cortisone preparations have many of the chemical actions of cortisol. They are, in fact, converted to cortisol in the body. I reasoned that if the endocrine-immune imbalance originated in an inadequate supply of cortisol, and that if therapeutic treatment with cortisone preparations reduced a significant degree of clinical signs, at least in the short term, perhaps smaller, long-term physiological doses of cortisone rather than the large, conventional pharmaceutical doses might be effective in regulating the condition long-term. In human medicine, William Jefferies, M.D., emeritus clinical professor of internal medicine at the University of Virginia, has treated humans for decades using this approach and reported improvement among patients with allergies, autoimmune disorders, and chronic fatigue.[1]

Over time I developed a testing and treatment strategy that proved to be safe and highly effective. The central modality is replacement of the cortisol deficiency/defect with physiological doses of various cortisone preparations. This normalizes the activity of ACTH, stops the overproduction of adrenal estrogen and the blockage of thyroid, and re-regulates the immune system. A second important modality is the simultaneous use of thyroid hormone. This is necessary in all canine cases, and in about 10 percent of feline cases. The contrasting thyroid requirement between dogs and cats is an apparent species-specific variation.

Elevated estrogen causes a binding effect on thyroid hormone resulting in retarded metabolic activity, impairing detoxification and the liver's ability to process the cortisol replacement. In this situation, even physiologic doses of cortisone may accumulate in the body and create side effects. By giving cortisol and thyroid replacement simultaneously, the body is able to effectively utilize the cortisol without side effects developing.

Once the hormone imbalance has been identified through the testing procedure described below, it is of paramount importance to initiate a hypoallergenic diet at the same time the hormone replacement program is started. The combination of daily feeding a commercial pet food, which typically has poor quality ingredients, and deregulated IgA in the digestive tract often leads to malabsorption and food allergies. The therapy program will not succeed if animals continue eating food to which they are sensitive. Within a few weeks, as animals improve on the program, pet owners can introduce different foods back into the diet one at a time, but should stay alert for signs of sensitivity to specific foods.

In the late 1970s, I wrote a series of reports in veterinary journals describing my findings and protocols.[2] As I uncovered these biochemical complexities in my research, I found no germane research in veterinary medicine to provide guidance. To my knowledge, the comprehensive endocrine-immune abnormality described here has not been reported elsewhere in major veterinary endocrine texts. However, many other genetic disorders among purebred pets, a result of contemporary breeding practices, have been reported.[3]

In the beginning, the flawed endocrine-immune mechanism appeared to be involved as an aggravating factor, that is, exacerbating allergies and sensitivities to food and parasites such as fleas. But with time, and a proliferation of breed-specific animals, gene pools have become narrower and narrower. I have consistently identified this mechanism in overt life-threatening diseases like severe autoimmunity and cancer, as have other veterinarians using this approach. It appears not only to cause typical allergy problems but because of its deregulating impact on the immune system also sets the stage for killer diseases. Younger animals with the defect are developing diseases previously seen only in older animals. Moreover, it often causes not just one illness but multiple disorders.

Research and clinical outcomes clearly identify this mechanism as a major factor in the etiology of common diseases. Associated diseases and disorders include malabsorption and digestive disorders, allergies, lung and urinary tract problems, sluggish liver function, strange or aggressive behavior, epilepsy, obesity, deadly viral and bacterial infections, periodontitis, vaccinosis, autoimmunity, and cancer.

The endocrine-immune derangement is not limited to purebreds. Affected purebreds have mated with mixed breeds until the mechanism is now widely established among both groups. I now find formerly breed-specific disorders appearing in other breeds as well as in mixed breeds.

While genetics appears to be the overwhelming cause of the imbalance, environmental factors such as food intolerance, poor diet, sensitivities to parasites, pollution, stress, and aging also enter into the equation.

Whatever the original cause, correction of the defect with appropriate levels of cortisone, thyroid and other hormones as needed in a long-term hormone replacement and therapy program consistently helps even severely diseased animals to live long and healthy lives.

The therapy does not cure. It funds a deficit, realigns a hormonal derangement, resets the metabolism, and restores normalcy to a dysfunctional immune system. It controls disease and supports the health of the animal for as long as the program is maintained. When pet owners stop the therapy, animals deteriorate and signs of previous illness return.

I have personally treated thousands of dogs and cats with this approach. As I write this, about two hundred other veterinarians are successfully using the program in the U.S. and elsewhere.

I have also worked with interested equine veterinarians and breeders and found a widespread endocrine-immune defect present in horses. Many common equine ailments have been corrected using the criteria described here. In the case of horses, most respond to thyroid replacement alone, while a few require both thyroid and cortisol.

The volume of global clinical experience clearly indicates that animals who might otherwise be destined for euthanasia or a life of suffering can be effectively tested and treated. It is also clear that the endocrine-immune test described below can be used preventively to determine the presence of imbalance even in asymptomatic animals.

Though it is beyond my capacity as a clinician to explore the molecular details of this widespread yet overlooked problem, a thorough investigation into its genetic and biochemical nature is clearly warranted.

TESTING FOR THE ENDOCRINE-IMMUNE IMBALANCE

I have developed a test that measures a critical range of hormonal and immune relationships: cortisol, total estrogen, T3, T4, IgA, IgM, and IgG, and therefore the impact of the HPA axis on the immune system. Cortisol itself, even if the value is normal, may be partially or completely bound (inactive) due to the nature of the genetic defect. Therefore, looking at the cortisol-estrogen-immunoglobulin relationship is essential. A cortisol problem likely exists if the estrogen level is high and the immunoglobulins are low.

The test is available to veterinarians through National Veterinary Diagnostic Services in Lake Forest, California. Veterinarians do not routinely utilize comprehensive tests such as these. They tend not to measure these levels and often prescribe steroids that may be too strong or not appropriate, a practice that frequently results in side effects.

Standard tests measure only one component of estrogen—estradiol. Total estrogen is a more accurate measurement because various estrogen compounds may be present in varying quantities. Estrogen can exert a dramatic blocking effect on cortisol and thyroid hormones; just a slight variation out of the normal range is enough to cause hormonal and immune complications. Elevated estrogen can bind thyroid hormone, rendering it partially or totally inactive, slowing overall metabolism, and triggering additional problems in the body. Much of the thyroid hormone in the body may in fact be inactive even if thyroid values in the test are normal.

The critical value of this test to the clinician is that it offers a comparative view of endocrine-immune relationships. A singular hormone level found in the high normal range for one animal may be an inadequate level for another, while a low level for one animal might be too high for another. Each animal, like each human, is biochemically individual. Reading empirical levels alone without considering the relationship of one hormone to another or of one hormone to a body system is like "missing the forest for the trees," as the old expression has it. In this case, the relationships are usually low cortisol, high estrogen, and deregulated immune cells. If the hormonal values in this test fall into the normal range, but if the animal is chronically ill and the immune cells are low, the therapy approach is the same, only the practitioner would use even less cortisone and thyroid than usual. Retesting after two weeks provides a gauge for determining the efficacy of the therapy. If the immunoglobulin values increase, and symptoms decrease, the course it correct. This is usually what happens.

Earlier, I included T cell values in the panel and found that the defect described here also suppresses T cells. However, due to the significant added cost for this measurement, I dropped T cells from the blood test panel.

More than 90 percent of the cases I treat involve neutered animals. Thus, in the case of female animals, there is no influence of ovarian estrogen, only adrenal estrogen. Among the female dogs and cats with intact ovaries, testing and therapy are conducted when animals are not in estrus and not producing a high level of ovarian estrogen.

In summary, the test reveals this cascade of pathology-causing effects:

1. **The production of insufficient or inactive cortisol in the middle layer (zona fasiculata) of the adrenal cortex.** If the cortisol is in the normal range, it may be largely bound and therefore not available for the body's use. The presence of high estrogen and low immunoglobulins indicate that the cortisol is inactive.

2. **The presence of elevated estrogen, a result of stimulation of the inner cortical layer (zona reticularis) where adrenal estrogen is produced.** There is no relationship to cyclic ovarian production of estrogen. In about 5 percent to 7 percent of cases, the zona reticularis appears to be also defective, that is, unable to produce adequate estrogen. In this situation, the animal, in essence, has a two-layer adrenal defect. This can, and does, contribute to the sequence of reduced immune regulation.

3. **Binding of thyroid hormone.** This estrogenic effect can be ascertained by the following signs when both T3 and T4 test normal: excess sleeping; sluggishness; hyperkeratosis of the nose and pads of feet; excess pigmentation in skin of ventral abdomen; high cholesterol (not diet related); high triglycerides (not diet related); no increase in body weight; many patients are actually underweight.

4. **A major deregulation and suppression of IgA, IgM, and IgG.**

Animals are retested after two weeks and again at subsequent intervals, depending on the seriousness of the condition. Although improvements occur rapidly after a hormone replacement program is initiated, retesting serves as a yardstick to gauge progress, evaluate normalizing endocrine-immune relationships, and consider possible adjustments in medication. I use a combination of pharmaceutical and plant-based cortisone preparations for patients, depending on the severity of disease.

True genetic imbalances require life-long management. Acquired imbalances can occur as a result of stress or exposure to toxic chemicals, anesthesia, heavy metals, or pollutants. They may require only temporary management but in some cases a lifetime of replacement therapy may be needed if symptoms return after therapy is discontinued.

Application for Humans

Does this clinical research and therapy offer similar promise for humans? Can cancer in humans be treated this way? I find the imbalance present in *every* animal cancer case I have treat. Treatment outcomes are usually positive, even in advanced cases.

Can AIDS be treated effectively with long-term cortisone replacement? Feline immunodeficiency virus (FIV) and human immunodeficiency virus (HIV) involve similar retroviral agents. I have achieved a 70 percent success rate in treating felines with symptomatic FIV. These animals remain disease-free as long as they remain on the hormone replacement program. When a human is exposed to the HIV virus, whether or not he or she develops AIDS may depend on whether the endocrine-immune system is in balance. If the system is normal, or has been normalized through replacement therapy, the virus may be fully neutralized and rendered incapable of "causing" disease. The virus, in fact, may not cause the disease but rather overwhelms a deregulated immune system. Therefore, the immune system's deregulation allows the disease.

Jefferies has reported in great detail on the safe and effective use of physiologic dosages of cortisone medication for a variety of human illnesses involving adrenocortical deficiency. This clinical perspective has been overlooked or dismissed by the vast majority of the medical community. In Jefferies' words, the reason relates to the "unique situation in which a normal hormone, one that is essential for life, has developed such a bad reputation that many physicians and patients are afraid to use it under any circumstances."[4] This reason probably applies as well to a similar situation in veterinary medicine.

Jefferies believes that indefinite replacement with physiologic dosages of cortisone will benefit many, if not all, patients with chronic allergies and autoimmune disorders, and that replacement should not be stopped upon initial remission.[5] My extensive experience treating sick animals clearly indicates that this is the right course of action. In the veterinary setting, if medication is stopped, the imbalance and symptoms return.

In the human setting, I would further suggest that clinicians should test patients for the same range of hormonal-immune relationships as I do for animals. That means a blood test to measure cortisol, total estrogen, thyroid (T3/T4), and immunoglobulins. Other measurements could be added, such as T cells and perhaps other hormones, in order to develop a more precise picture of the defect's total range of impact. Patients can be retested at biweekly or monthly intervals to monitor the changing hormone and immune relationships.

In the case of female patients, the clinician will have to take ovarian estrogen status into consideration. The level of total estrogen will change depending on the stage of the woman's menstrual cycle; whether or not she is pregnant; whether she is of reproductive age, perimenopausal or menopausal, or taking an estrogen replacement. A testing method will have to be structured that accommodates these individual situations. One approach for menstruating females might be to test in mid-cycle when the ovarian estrogen level is highest and again just prior to menses when it is at the lowest level, subtract to find the difference, and use that as a basis for determining non-ovarian estrogen values. The calculated non-ovarian estrogen values could then be used for comparison with immune cell values.

In addition, the clinician might want to obtain a 24-hour urine sample from the patient in order to test for active T3, T4, and cortisol. This would be an important diagnostic tool allowing a comparison to blood values, which may test out as normal but in fact may involve a significant percentage of bound (inactive) hormones.

The other limitation of testing blood levels alone relates to the possible presence of a sluggish metabolism. In such a situation blood levels may be higher or normal because of the retarded speed of processing within the system. Growing numbers of physicians are becoming aware that hypothyroidism may exist even though thyroid blood levels appear normal. Again, the urine test can help clarify this issue.

As in veterinary medicine, little is known regarding cortisol deficiency states in humans. Jefferies suggests that mild degrees of deficiency may be due either to primary adrenal malfunction or secondary to inadequate stimulation by the pituitary or hypothalamus. One should mention the pioneering work of Hans Selye, who demonstrated that cortisol deficiency is a clear consequence of prolonged stress and contributes to some of the "diseases of civilization."[6]

The role genetics plays in humans is unknown. One can only speculate that an adrenal or cortisol defect could be passed on to offspring if, both parents are affected.

If the imbalance becomes expressed in children, could perhaps the impact of deregulated IgA create widespread loss of critical immunity in mucous tissue throughout the body? The effect could possibly create one or more of the following conditions: allergies, hay fever, asthma, food sensitivities, malabsorption, or digestive tract, bladder, kidney and lung problems. Testing for the imbalance and correcting the cortisol defect, if it exists, could perhaps circumvent the development of chronic health disorders in children. Among young girls, it might be easier to determine a damaging influence from adrenal estrogen at an age before ovarian estrogen is present.

I have seen an escalating severity of conditions related to this defect in generations of animals. Is there a parallel development among humans? Can we expect to see allergies and malabsorption in one generation, and an increased potential for more serious conditions like autoimmune diseases and cancer?

These are all issues to be explored once the mechanism in humans has been identified.

CONCLUSION

The role of cortisol as an immune regulatory agent has been grossly neglected. An unknown but probably very large percentage of sick cats and dogs produce inadequate or bound cortisol as a result of contemporary breeding practices and, to a lesser degree, stress, aging, poor diet, and other environmental factors. The cortisol defect triggers a chain of biochemical events that results in elevated estrogen, bound thyroid hormone, and deregulation of major immune system cells. I have treated thousands of pets with a wide variety of otherwise intractable health problems by correcting this endocrine-immune abnormality with a hormone replacement program.

The program consists of physiologic doses of cortisone plus thyroid replacement in dogs, and cortisone alone in most cases for cats. Continued for the long-term over the course of an animal's life, this approach effectively controls even severe diseases and contributes to health and longevity.

A test to determine the presence of the imbalance has been described, and can serve veterinarians as an important diagnostic tool for a potentially deadly yet overlooked cause of disease. The test also serves conscientious breeders to determine the health status of breeding stock and whether certain animals should be bred or not. The rationale here is that use of this test by breeders can help to reverse an alarming rise in genetically based pathology that threatens the survival of domesticated canines and felines.

It is my belief that a similar hormonal-immune sequence is a common, yet largely overlooked factor in human pathology and should be investigated. Jefferies has reported that physiologic dosages of cortisone can improve a number of human disorders involving an adrenocortical deficiency. His work has been largely overlooked. The experience with animals and the work of Jefferies and his followers strongly argues for exploring this area that may produce major diagnostic and treatment breakthroughs.

REFERENCES

1. Jefferies, W. McK. Mild adrenocortical deficiency, chronic allergies, autoimmune disorders and the chronic fatigue syndrome: A continuation of the cortisone story. *Medical Hypotheses,* 1994; 42: 183-189.

2. Plechner A. J., Shannon, M. Canine immune complex diseases. *Modern Veterinary Practice,* November 1976: 917.

3. Lemonick, M. D. A Terrible Beauty: An obsessive focus on show-ring looks is crippling, sometimes fatally, America's purebred dogs. *Time,* December 12, 1994: 65.

4. Jefferies, op. cit., 185.

5. Jefferies, op. cit., 188.

6. Selye, H. Studies on adaptation. *Endocrinology,* 1937, 21: 169.

Adrenal-Immune Disturbance in Animals Offers Therapeutic Insights for Multiple Human Disorders

©Alfred J. Plechner, D.V.M.
Originally published in *Townsend Letter for Doctors & Patients*, as "Chaos in the Cortex," April 2003

In thousands of cases spanning three decades, I have identified an unrecognized endocrine-immune disturbance as a major trigger of multiple disorders in dogs and cats, including allergies, epilepsy, viral diseases, inflammatory bowel, autoimmunity, and cancer. In most cases, and for seemingly unrelated conditions, I have restored health by correcting this disturbance with the same therapeutic program.

I strongly believe this clinical approach offers important diagnostic and treatment promise for common human diseases that may also have a similar mechanism of endocrine-immune imbalance.

The problem originates with genetic or acquired disturbance to the adrenal cortex production of cortisol. A domino effect ensues, affecting the hypothalamus-pituitary-adrenal axis. Estrogen, from the apparent conversion of adrenal androgens, is overproduced. Thyroid hormones are blocked. Immune function becomes compromised. I consistently see this scenario in sick patients, and *every* cancer patient I treat has it.

CLINICAL EVOLUTION

Early in my career I realized I was just providing temporary relief for most of my patients. I was practicing what I had been taught in veterinary school, but I was merely treating medical effects, and doing no real healing. I felt frustrated. I wanted to make a difference in the health of my patients. So I embarked on a personal mission to better understand the causes of sickness.

The process started in 1969 when a medical research laboratory contracted me to inspect their animal-testing environment. Instead of a fee I asked the laboratory to run antibody levels on my patients. I did this to develop a better sense of immune function in relation to norms, disease, and effects of treatment. The laboratory monitored five immunoglobulins for me: IgA, IgD, IgE, IgG, and IgM.

After two years I was able to define normal and abnormal ranges for what I considered the most significant antibodies relating to viruses, bacteria, fungal conditions, and hypersensitivity. For me, the most relevant antibodies were IgG, IgM, and, in particular, IgA.

I first applied these standards to Sunshine, a very sick Golden Retriever puppy. The young dog had a serious autoimmune-like problem with horrible inflamed skin. Antibody levels were quite low. I prescribed a standard daily dosage of cortisone to reduce the inflammation and an antibiotic to handle the bacteria. Within a few days the dog was much better.

I retested for antibodies and was shocked. The antibodies were clearly improved from baseline levels before treatment.

How could this occur? I had expected the anti-inflammatory effect. After all, cortisone is used for that purpose. But everybody knows (or at least believes) that cortisone suppresses immune cells. So why did the antibodies increase?

I started reading physiology and endocrinology books seeking an explanation. I found basic information, but no explanation.

I learned that cortisol, the primary adrenal glucocorticoid hormone produced in the middle cortex layer (zona fasciculata), exerts an anti-inflammatory effect. This action inspired the development of cortisone (synthetic cortisol) drugs. Cortisol also serves as a "stress hormone," causing the release of glucose to fuel a response to danger. Less understood is its role as a regulator of the immune system. Cortisol is stimulated by the pituitary's adrenocorticotropic hormone (ACTH), which, in turn, is controlled by the hypothalamic corticotropic-releasing factor (CRF). Secretion is governed by a classical feedback loop. When blood concentrations rise to a certain level, cortisol inhibits CRF secretion. This then inhibits ACTH and cortisol secretion.

I learned that when the zona fasciculata cannot make enough cortisol, or for some reason the cortisol is excessively bound (inactive) or defective and thus not recognized by the system, the pituitary continues to release ACTH in order to stimulate more cortisol. Somehow this results in elevated estrogen in the body.

I wondered if a physiologically significant amount of estrogen could be pushed into the system by abnormal adrenal-hypothalamus-pituitary activity stemming from a cortisol defect or deficiency. Could this added estrogen contribute to inflammation? The research says that estrogen stimulates histamine release. Histamine causes inflammation. Could cortisone medication correct a cortisol deficiency, turn off the ACTH demand, and reduce the adrenal stimulation of estrogen? Could this help explain in part why cortisone so effectively brings down inflammation?

The questions piled up. Over time, and with continued clinical investigation, the practical answers came that enabled me to effectively test and treat my patients.

In sick animals I consistently found low cortisol, high estrogen (no matter whether the animal was male, female, or neutered), and low antibodies. Repeated testing showed the same hormonal imbalance coinciding with abnormal levels of IgA, IgG, and IgM antibodies. The result, in case after case: poor resistance against viral, bacterial, and fungal infections and a greater susceptibility to disease.

I found that cortisone therapy initially lowers estrogen and increases antibody levels. Continued cortisone usage, however, causes antibodies to fall again—an immunosuppressive effect that occurs even with very low cortisone dosages. Eventually, I came to the conclusion that the elevated estrogen must be binding thyroid hormones, thus slowing the metabolism and the body's ability to process the cortisone. Even if blood tests showed thyroid to be "normal," estrogen was invariably high and antibodies low. Moreover, I would often find slower than normal heart rate, lower than normal temperature, and higher than normal levels of cholesterol and triglycerides, all markers of a thyroid problem.

If I treated dogs simultaneously with cortisone and thyroid hormone, the estrogen level decreased and the antibodies increased and stayed in the normal immunocompetence range. Canine patients improved. They seemed to process the cortisone and disallow toxic buildup. For some species-specific reason, most cats needed only the cortisone, not the thyroid.

I eventually figured out effective dosages of cortisone replacement that worked both therapeutically and for long-term use without side effects. These levels of dosages turned out to be physiologic, that is, significantly lower than conventional pharmacologic levels. The low dosages lower estrogen and increase antibodies. In my therapy program, I utilize a combination of pharmaceutical and plant-based (natural) cortisone preparations, depending on the severity and stage of disease. Many once-sick animals have been on this program for their entire lifetimes and remained healthy.

For years I thought that the inner cortex layer, called the zona reticularis and which also responds to ACTH, produced estrogen. I later learned that this zone produces the androgens dehydroepiandrosterone (DHEA) and dehydroepiandrosterone sulfate (DHEAS), the most abundant circulating hormones in the body. These substances are known as prohormones in that they metabolize into other hormones. Through enzymatic actions they can convert to androstenedione, androstenediol, testosterone, and further to the estrogen compounds estrone and estradiol. Androstenedione, for instance, is the main precursor of estrone, the most abundant circulating estrogen in postmenopausal women. Androstenediol, converted from DHEA, has inherent estrogenic activity.[1] I believe these androgen-to-estrogen processes may be producing the elevated estrogen.

Causes of an Epidemic

In thousands of cases I have repeatedly observed the same endocrine-immune dysfunction operating. It undermines homeostasis and sets the stage for malabsorption and digestive disorders, allergies, lung and urinary tract problems, sluggish liver function, strange or aggressive behavior, epilepsy, obesity, deadly viral and bacterial infections, periodontitis, vaccine reactions, autoimmunity, and cancer. Younger animals with the defect develop diseases typically seen in older animals. Moreover, the defect often causes not just one illness, but multiple illnesses.

I consider the problem in pets to be largely genetic. Early on, I observed similar problems among littermates and along familial lines: severe hypersensitivity, inflamed skin with ulcerations and itchiness, malabsorption, and internal systems seemingly out of control. I began to suspect that contemporary breeding practices—namely inbreeding and linebreeding for a fashionable appearance instead of for function and hardiness—were causing narrowed gene pools, compromised health, and shortened longevity. Many genetic disorders among purebred pets, a result of contemporary breeding practices, have been reported.[2] However, other than my published papers, the endocrine-immune abnormality described here has not been reported.

The abnormality goes beyond purebreds. As affected purebreds have mated with mixed breeds the defect has proliferated. I believe it is extremely widespread and an unrecognized cause of the disease epidemic among household pets.

Food intolerances, poor diet, sensitivities to parasites, stress, and aging, also enter into the equation. Environmental toxicity could be another significant, yet largely unrecognized, factor. It is generally recognized adrenal gland is the most vulnerable organ in the endocrine system for toxins, and within the adrenal gland "the majority of effects" have been observed in the cortex. Such disturbances can "fundamentally affect the whole body physiology and biochemistry."[3]

Whatever the original cause, correction of the disturbance with appropriate low-dosage cortisone (along with thyroid replacement in dogs) generally restores immunocompetence and health. Even severely diseased animals make comebacks, living long and healthy lives. But animals deteriorate when pet owners, for whatever reason, stop the therapy. Signs of previous illness return. The treatment funds a deficit, realigns a hormonal derangement, resets the metabolism, and restores coherence to an incoherent immune system. It controls disease and supports the health of the animal for as long as the program is maintained. Used therapeutically, it can save animals who might otherwise be destined for euthanasia. Used preventively to determine the presence of imbalance in asymptomatic animals, it can help avoid future suffering and premature death.

IS THIS CONGENITAL ADRENAL HYPERPLASIA?

I have found nothing in the medical literature—veterinary or human—exactly describing this endocrine-immune pattern and and its broad medical effects. Congenital adrenal hyperplasia (CAH) has some similarities. This human condition is characterized by a deficiency of cortisol and an increase in androgens, the result of a deficiency in the adrenal enzymes that make cortisol. Once considered a rare inherited disorder with severe manifestations, a mild form is now said to be common although frequently undiagnosed. Patients with the mild form are fre-

quently unable to mount sufficient stress responses to trauma and infection.[4]

It is possible that a similar enzyme disturbance could be operating in household pets. I have not tested for enzyme deficiencies or for androgen levels.

There are at least two clear dissimilarities between CAH and the endocrine-immune defect I have identified in animals. CAH involves hypertrophy of the adrenal glands and frequent deficiency of aldosterone, the mineralocorticoid produced by the outer layer of the cortex. I have neither in affected animals.

I am a clinician, not a researcher. I have learned what I know first-hand from testing and treating my patients over many years. Looking back, I was very fortunate to uncover a therapeutic path that has worked magnificently. While researchers now recognize that the hypothalamic-pituitary-adrenal axis, as part of the neuroendocrine system, has central importance to immune homeostasis,[5] they still admit to a lack of clear understanding about countless details and interactions.

TESTING FOR THE MECHANISM

Years ago I developed a special blood test to monitor the key hormonal and immune levels and relationships for cortisol, total estrogen, T3, T4, IgA, IgM, and IgG. The reference ranges evolved from clinical observation in thousands of cases. Comprehensive tests such as these are not utilized routinely by veterinarians.

An initial test gives me baselines before therapy starts. High estrogen and low antibodies are the major clues I look for. Two weeks after therapy begins I retest to see how values have shifted and adjust the program accordingly. Once values normalize and clinical signs abate, I retest on a six-month or annual basis.

I compare hormone relationships to each other and to the immune system, rather than relying on individual levels. Cortisol itself, even if the value is normal, may be in a bound (inactive) state to some degree due to the nature of the cortical defect. T3/T4 could show normal, but also be bound. Moreover, a singular hormone level found in the high normal range for one animal could be an inadequate level for another, while a low level for one animal might be too high for another. For these reasons I compare the range of test values with clinical signs. Generally, I look to bring down total estrogen, raise antibodies, and free up T3/T4. This typically parallels a clinical improvement in the patient.

Earlier, I included T cell testing and found that the mechanism also suppresses T cells. However, due to the significant added cost, I dropped T cell measurement from the panel.

Standard tests measure only one estrogen compound: estradiol. I test for total estrogen, that is, all the estrogen compounds in the body. I feel this is a more accurate indicator because of the potential for the estrogens to exert a blocking effect on cortisol and thyroid. Just a slight variation out of normal is enough to disturb hormonal and immune activity. As I mentioned earlier, elevated estrogen binds thyroid hormones to a varying degree, enough to slow down overall metabolism, and trigger additional problems.

About 90 percent of my cases involve neutered animals. Thus, in the case of spayed females, and males (intact or otherwise), I attribute the high estrogen level to probable androgen-to-estrogen conversion. Testing of female dogs and cats with intact ovaries is conducted when animals are not not in estrus, and therefore not producing a high level of ovarian estrogen.

APPLICATION FOR HUMANS

Does this endocrine-immune disturbance exist in humans? And if so, can a similar treatment protocol be applied?

I have suggested to interested physicians that they test their human patients for the same range of hormonal-immune relationships that I test in my animal patients. That means a blood test measuring cortisol, total estrogen, thyroid (T3/T4), and immunoglobulins. Other factors could be added, such as T cells and the androgen precursors to estrogen, in order to develop a more precise picture. Researchers have begun looking at the immune and inflammatory modulating effects of androgen/estrogen ratios and concentrations.[6]

Patients can be retested at biweekly or monthly intervals to monitor changing relationships. The bottom line is that hormonal replacement must be measured against B and T cell levels.

For female patients, clinicians will have to consider ovarian estrogen. The level of total estrogen will obviously vary according to the stage of the monthly cycle at which testing is done, age, and use of birth control pills or estrogen replacement. Reproductive age females might be tested in mid-cycle when the ovarian estrogen level is highest and again just prior to menses when it is

at the lowest level. Reproductive-age women should be tested on the seventh day of the cycle, when estrogen is lowest, and again on the twenty first day, when estrogen is highest. The difference between the two scores should reflect non-ovarian estrogen in the system. One physician who uses hormones routinely in his practice was surprised to find, after I discussed this mechanism with him, that his sickest postmenopausal (non-ERT) patients had high estrogen levels and low antibody counts. The possible reason for this, I suggested, is the impact of low/bound cortisol and added estrogen from adrenal androgen conversion. Estrogen synthesis is known to increase in non-ovarian tissues as a function of age and body weight.[7] Even though postmenopausal, these women may actually be in a state of relative estrogen dominance.

The clinician might also want to obtain a 24-hour urine sample from the patient in order to test for active T3, T4, cortisol, total estrogen, and any other relevant markers. This would allow a comparison to blood values, which may test out as normal but in fact involve significantly bound hormones. Often it is not known if the hormone is working or not. The urine test can help answer this question and contribute to a more effective treatment.

Can a comprehensive endocrine-immune strategy help human cancer patients? The imbalance exists in each and every animal cancer case referred to me. Therapy outcomes are usually positive, even in advanced cases when hormone replacement therapy is combined with excision, chemotherapy, or radiation.

What about AIDS? In cats, the feline immunodeficiency virus (FIV) involves a retrovirus similar to HIV. Veterinarians put down symptomatic cats, yet I have a 70 percent recovery rate among such patients. They remain disease-free as long as they are maintained on low-dosage cortisone. Cats testing positive for the virus do not develop clinical signs once they go on—and stay on—the program. I suggest that when a human is exposed to the HIV virus, whether or not he or she develops symptoms of AIDS may depend on the strength of his or her endocrine-immune connections. If an imbalance is found through testing, correction with appropriate hormone replacement could be a significant strategy for both prevention and therapy.

Can this mechanism contribute to human inflammatory bowel conditions such as colitis and Crohn's disease? There is currently an epidemic of inflammatory gut conditions among dogs and cats. I consistently find the imbalance in affected animals. The therapy works well. The typical low cortisol/high estrogen combination destabilizes and depletes IgA, a global antibody most active in the mucous membranes of the body, including the gut lining. Low IgA suggests an absorption problem. The animal (or human) may not absorb oral medication, so I begin therapy with intramuscular injections of cortisone, or, in the case of life-threatening conditions, intravenous drips, along with thyroid replacement and a hypoallergenic diet, which minimizes the risk of food-related reactions. This total approach quickly lowers the estrogen level and raises IgA. Once IgA rises to a certain point and the inflammation has subsided, I switch to oral medication. The same approach works for IgA-related conditions elsewhere. Animals with chronic bowel disorders (including food allergies), respiratory and urinary tract disorders, and anaphylactic and vaccine reactions invariably have abnormal IgA levels.

William Jefferies, M.D., of the University of Virginia, has described the safe and effective use of physiologic dosages of cortisone for decades in human patients with "adrenocortical deficiency."[8] He has reported improvement among patients with allergies, autoimmune disorders, and chronic fatigue[9] yet the medical community has largely ignored his research. The reason, he states, relates to the "unique situation in which a normal hormone, one that is essential for life, has developed such a bad reputation that many physicians and patients are afraid to use it under any circumstances."[10] This comment accurately describes my experience in veterinary medicine. At pharmacologic dosages, cortisone does indeed create side effects. Practitioners shudder at any suggestion of long-term cortisone, even small physiologic dosages acting as a hormone replacement for deficient cortisol.

Jefferies believes that replacement with physiologic dosages of cortisone should not be stopped upon initial remission.[11] I agree. In my experience with animals, stopping the medication virtually guarantees that the imbalance and its secondary clinical signs will return.

SUMMING IT UP

I have found nothing in the literature to fully documenting the devastating effects of deficient or bound cortisol and elevated estrogen on the immune systems of household pets.

Animals born with defective adrenal glands eventually get sick. One can speculate that a cortisol defect could be passed on to offspring if both parents are affected. This appears to be a widespread problem among cats and dogs. I have seen an escalating severity of conditions related to this defect in generations of animals.

Is there a parallel development among humans with allergies and malabsorption in one generation and autoimmune diseases and cancer in the next?

Stress, poor diet and environmental toxins are other possible explanations for adrenal malfunction. Hans Selye's seminal work in 1937 demonstrated that cortisol deficiency is a clear consequence of prolonged stress and contributes to some of the "diseases of civilization."[12]

Jefferies' excellent work examines the effects of mild cortisol deficiency due to either primary adrenal malfunction or secondary to inadequate stimulation by the pituitary or hypothalamus. He has reported that physiologic dosages of cortisone can improve a number of human disorders.

Recently, other medical researchers have reported successful applications of low dosage cortisone in rheumatoid arthritis and polymyalgia rheumatica, a systemic inflammatory disorder of the aged.[13, 14] CAH is treated, in part, with cortisone replacement.[15] The resemblance between adrenal defects in animals and CAH in humans strongly suggests that comparative research is warranted.

My independent clinical experience shows that low-dose cortisone, along with thyroid replacement, helps restore lost immune competence in many dogs. In most affected cats, cortisol alone works. I have learned that hormones regulate the immune system and when I normalize the key hormones I can usually restore immune competence and health to my patients.

Open-minded veterinarians who have inquired about this approach and applied it in their practices have obtained similar results. It has not been tested, however, in controlled studies. Nor has it been studied in humans. As a clinician I cannot carry out the elaborate research necessary to fully explore this largely unrecognized condition, but I believe such research could produce major diagnostic and treatment breakthroughs for humans.

REFERENCES

1. Parker, L. N. Adrenal androgens. In *Endocrinology* (Ed: DeGroot), Third Edition, Philadelphia: W. B. Saunders Co., 1995: 1836-47.

2. Lemonick M. D. A Terrible Beauty: An obsessive focus on show-ring looks is crippling, sometimes fatally, America's purebred dogs. *Time,* December 12, 1994: ; 65.

3. Harvey P. W. *The Adrenal in Toxicology: Target Organ and Modulator of Toxicity,* Bristol, PA (Taylor & Francis), 1996: 7.

4. Deaton, M., et al. Congenital adrenal hyperplasia: Not really a zebra. *American Family Physician,* March 1, 1999: 1190.

5. Cutolo M, et al. Altered neuroendocrine immune (NEI) networks in rheumatology. *Annals of the New York Academy of Sciences,* June 2002, 966: xvii.

6. Cutolo M., et al. Androgens and estrogens modulate the immune and inflammatory responses in rheumatoid arthritis. *Annals of the New York Academy of Sciences,* June 2002, 966: 131-142.

7. Gruber, C. J., et al. Production and actions of estrogens. *New England Journal of Medicine,* 2002, 346 (5): 340-52).

8. Jefferies W. McK. *Safe Uses of Cortisol.* Springfield, IL (Charles C. Thomas Publisher), 1996.

9. Jefferies W. McK. Mild adrenocortical deficiency, chronic allergies, autoimmune disorders and the chronic fatigue syndrome: A continuation of the cortisone story. *Medical Hypotheses,* 1994; 42; 183-189.

10. Jefferies, op. cit., 185.

11. Jefferies, op. cit., 188.

12. Selye, H. Studies on adaptation. *Endocrinology,* 1937, 21;: 169.

13. Hickling P., et al. Joint destruction after glucocorticoids are withdrawn in early rheumatoid arthritis. *British Journal of Rheumatology,* 1998; 37: 930-936.

14. Cutolo M., et al. Cortisol, dehydroepiandrosterone sulfate, and androstenedione levels in patients with polymyalgia rheumatica during twelve months of glucocorticoid therapy. *Annals of the New York Academy of Sciences,* June 2002, 966: 91-96.

15. Deaton, M., et al, op. cit., 1190.

Do Adrenal-Immune Disturbances in Animals and Common Variable Immunodeficiency in Humans Have a Common Cause?

©Alfred J. Plechner, D.V.M.

Letter to the editor, first published in *Townsend Letter for Doctors & Patients,* June 2003

In my April *Townsend Letter* article, "Chaos in the Cortex,"(titled "Unrecognized Adrenal-Immune Disturbance in Pets Offers Therapeutic Insights for Multiple Human Disorders" in this volume) I suggest that the endocrine-immune disturbance I have found in many thousands of canine and feline cases over thirty years of veterinary practice may offer insights for human medicine. Since writing that article I have uncovered striking similarities to immune deficiency syndromes in humans. Just like the generally unsuspected problem I consistently see in animals, common variable immunodeficiency (CVID) in humans is a prime example of a widely underdiagnosed "enabling" mechanism for a multiplicity of disorders such as chronic infections, autoimmune conditions, an increased risk of cancer, and poor response to immunization.

In animals, I long ago linked destabilization of the immune system to adrenal cortex dysfunction. Specifically, I traced a pattern starting with a deficiency or ineffectiveness of cortisol, which is produced by the cortex. This defect creates a chain of hormonal imbalances, including elevated estrogen and interference with thyroid, which leads in turn to systemic inflammation, metabolism slowdown, and suppressed immune activity. Both B and T cells are reduced to the point of immunoincompetency.

Researchers recognize that the hypothalamic-pituitary-adrenal axis, as part of the neuroendocrine system, has central importance to immune homeostasis, but don't yet have a clear understanding of its countless interactions. As a clinician, I certainly don't know the molecular background to all of this, but I do know what undermines the health of my patients and how to correct the problem and restore health. From my experience it is clear that certain hormones have a profound regulating influence on immune function, and when these hormones are out of balance the immune system is also out of balance.

In CVID in humans is characterized by low IgA, IgG, and IgM levels, just as in animals, and often there are also problems with T cell function. In humans, the precise trigger for such immune dysfunction is unknown. Researchers have not linked CVID or other so-called immunodeficiency mechanisms to hormones. I suggest that exploring this connection, and looking at cortisol activity, may generate major clues for diagnosis and treatment.

Cortisol is the primary secretion of the adrenal glands in dogs and humans. It is a pivotal anti-inflammatory hormone. It also promotes the release of glucose to fuel an emergency response to danger. According to Dartmouth's Allan Munck, an expert on cortisol, normal activity of this hormone is almost certainly required for proper immune response.

TOO MUCH OR TOO LITTLE CORTISOL A PROBLEM

Cortisol has gotten a bad reputation because it becomes elevated by stress. If it remains elevated for long the immune system, fertility, bones, weight, memory, and insulin activity can suffer. Cortisol deficiency, on the other hand, tends to be overlooked, though it can cause many problems. It has been suggested that if stress goes on too long, then adrenal production becomes "exhausted" and cortisol deficiency may occur. Adrenal deficits have been linked to chronic fatigue, allergies, and rheumatoid arthritis in humans.

Cortisol deficiency may also result from toxicity. Within the endocrine system the adrenal cortex is the most vulnerable target for toxic elements.

Certainly heredity plays a role. In dogs and cats, contemporary practices of inbreeding for a fashionable look have led to a plethora of genetic defects. Through testing, I have found that many very young animals already have a cortisol problem and a resultant endocrine-immune imbalance. If not corrected, this imbalance triggers illness. The more significant the imbalance, the more severe the problems. Milder imbalances combined with environmental factors can, over time, cause disease later in life. If one or both parents have imbalances most litter members will, also. In some cases of human CVID, multiple family members are deficient in one or more antibody types. One family member may have CVID while another has selective IgA deficiency.

CORRECTING THE IMBALANCE

My standard treatment for affected animals is to correct the original cortisol deficiency with a safe and effective program of long-term, low-dosage cortisone, using either synthetic or natural preparations as required. While many practitioners may shudder at the thought of long-term cortisone use, I have found that that if done correctly, and if used to correct a cortisol deficiency, cortisone works safely and extremely well. This has in fact been reported in the medical literature by William Jefferies, emeritus clinical professor of internal medicine at the University of Virginia, and more recently by researchers in connection with autoimmune conditions and sepsis. Most dogs also require thyroid medication, while cats, for some species-specific reason, do not. I have an extremely high success rate with this approach, even with animals who are severely ill. Usually this approach rapidly normalizes antibody levels and restores immunocompetency to patients. Patients remain healthy for as long as they are kept on the therapy.

Humans with CVID receive gammaglobulin treatment, which is said to almost always bring some degree of improvement. Some patients may require long-term antibiotics, something I have not found necessary in animals once the endocrine-immune imbalance is corrected. It would be interesting to see if the cortisol/cortisone approach offers greater effectiveness and symptom relief.

I have been lucky enough to uncover a major connection between hormones and the immune system, and develop an effective testing and treatment protocol

HUMAN AND ANIMAL IMMUNE DEFICIENCY SIMILARITIES

As the following analysis shows, there are many similarities between CVID and the endocrine-immune imbalance in pets. Originally thought to be rare, it is now regarded as common. In pets, the endocrine-immune disturbance is common, yet unsuspected and unrecognized to date by "official" veterinary medicine.

CHARACTERISTIC	CVID	AI IMBALANCE IN PETS
An interaction of genetic and environmental factors is involved.	X	X
Diagnosis is confirmed by low level of serum antibodies, usually IgA, IgG, and IgM.	X	X
Medical effects can develop at any age. Symptoms can be mild to severe.	X	X
Chronic or recurring infections.	X	X
Infections are most often caused by the same organisms that trigger comparable infections in immunocompetent hosts, however immuno-deficient patients develop infections as well from opportunistic organisms, even organisms of relatively low virulence.	X	X
Patients can also develop severe infections, or complications.	X	X
Patients commonly develop enlarged lymph nodes.	X	X
Patients may develop polyarthritis of one or more joints.	X	X
Patients may develop malabsorption.	X	X
Patients may develop inflammatory bowel disease and GI complaints including abdominal pain, bloating, nausea, vomiting, diarrhea, and weight loss.	X	X
Patients have low IgA blood levels	X	X
Infectious giardia, campylobacter, salmonellae, shigella, and rotavirus can become chronic and lead to significant, even catastrophic weight loss.	X	X
A subgroup of up to 30 percent of human patients develop autoimmune conditions such as immune thrombocytopenic purpura, autoimmune hemolytic anemia, rheumatoid arthritis, lupus, autoimmune thyroiditis, or primary biliary cirrhosis. In animals I see these same conditions as well as pemphigus.	X	X
Patients can develop endocrine disorders such as thyroid disease or diabetes. Most canine patients have a primary or secondary thyroid imbalance.	X	X
Increased risk of cancer, particularly cancer of the lymph system, skin, and GI tract (in humans). In animals, all cancer patients, with all types of cancer, have an underlying endocrine-immune imbalance.	X	X
Immunizations usually produce very low or absent antibody levels.	X	X

that works magnificently for a broad spectrum of chronic and catastrophic diseases. I hope that this clinical experience may serve in the quest to understand, prevent, and treat human illnesses. I believe that the immune deficiency mechanism I have found in animals exists in some similar form in humans, and represents an extremely significant and insidious primer for disease.

I have begun to work with physicians interested in exploring the endocrine-immune approach to disease. I hope such contacts will expand, and that by sharing information and working together we can reduce the enormous burden of chronic disease that affects our society.

Cortisol Abnormality as a Cause of Elevated Estrogen and Immune Destabilization

©Alfred J. Plechner, D.V.M.
To be published in *Medical Hypotheses,* 2003

I have long regarded adrenal dysfunction as a well-spring of excess estrogen which may contribute to hormonal imbalances, immune destabilization, and increased vulnerability to disease. As a practicing clinician, I have consistently found elevated total estrogen as part of an endocrine-immune derangement present in many common diseases of dogs and cats. Ninety percent of these cases involve spayed females and neutered or intact males, so the elevated estrogen cannot be attributed to ovarian activity. Sick and intact females, tested outside their estrus period, frequently have an elevated estrogen level as well.

The pattern of derangement identified in thousands of cases over three decades involves insufficient cortisol, high estrogen, and abnormally low IgA, IgG, and IgM levels. This pattern undermines homeostasis and sets the stage for malabsorption and digestive disorders, allergies, lung and urinary tract problems, sluggish liver function, strange or aggressive behavior, epilepsy, obesity, deadly viral and bacterial infections, periodontitis, vaccine complications, autoimmunity, and cancer. Moreover, the same set of imbalances is often present as an underlying enabling mechanism in multiple illnesses.

The adrenal cortex produces a variety of vital hormones. Among them is cortisol, the primary glucocorticoid made in the middle cortex layer (zona fasciculata). Endogenous cortisol controls inflammation,[1] a function that inspired the development of cortisone drugs, pharmaceutical versions of cortisol. A profound loss of cortisol can lead to a critical state of deranged metabolism and an inability to deal with stress and infections. Cortisol exerts a discriminating regulatory effect on molecular mediators. These mediators trigger activity related to both immunity and inflammation. A normal level of cortisol seems to be required for healthy responses.[2] Cortisol deficiency may result in an unresponsive immune system, whereas too much cortisol—like too much cortisone medication—suppresses immune responses.

Adrenocorticotropic hormone (ACTH) from the pituitary stimulates cortisol production. ACTH is controlled in turn by the hypothalamic corticotropic-releasing factor (CRF) in a classical feedback loop. When cortisol blood concentrations rise to a certain level, CRF secretion slows, inhibiting ACTH and subsequent cortisol secretion.

The androgens dehydroepiandrosterone (DHEA) and dehydroepiandrosterone sulfate (DHEAS) are the most abundant circulating hormones in the body. These substances, known as prohormones because they metabolize into other hormones, are primarily made in the zona reticularis of the adrenal cortex. Through enzymatic actions, they convert to androstenedione, androstenediol, testosterone, and further to the estrogen compounds estrone and estradiol.[3] Androstenedione is the most important precursor of estrone, the most abundant circulating estrogen in postmenopausal women. Androstenediol has inherent estrogenic activity.[4]

The exact biological function of adrenal androgens and the mechanisms underlying their control is still the object of debate. However, it is well known that both may have androgenic and estrogenic effects.[5]

Veterinary researchers have found numerous genetic defects resulting from contemporary linebreeding and inbreeding practices.[6] Since the 1970s I have reported a cortisol defect in cats and dogs.[7] I believe this stems largely from questionable breeding practices.

Other potential causes for cortisol deficiency include prolonged stress and toxicity, which may be a significant acquired cause of adrenal cortical dysfunction. Harvey states that the adrenal gland is the most vulnerable organ in the endocrine system for toxins, and within the adrenal gland "the majority of effects" have been observed in the cortex. Such disturbances can "fundamentally affect the whole body physiology and biochemistry."[8]

When the zona fasciculata cannot make enough cortisol, or for some reason the cortisol is excessively bound (inactive) and thus not recognized by the hypothalamus-pituitary system, the pituitary continues to release ACTH in order to stimulate more cortisol. The zona reticularis also responds to ACTH. This part of the adrenal gland, as noted above, produces androgens that can convert to the estrogen compound estrone, or to testosterone, which may then convert in part to the more potent estrogen compound estradiol.

Some researchers say that an interface or transition zone of tissue between the zona fasciculata and reticularis of the adrenal cortex is capable of directly producing sex hormones, including estrogen compounds.[9, 10] Excess estrogen promotes CRF release from the hypothalamus and ACTH from the pituitary, and contributes to hormonal imbalances and deleterious effects in the body.

Researchers working in the field of rheumatoid arthritis and autoimmune rheumatic diseases believe that hormone balance is a crucial factor in the regulation of immune and inflammatory responses. Generally, estrogen in physiologic concentrations enhances humoral immune responses and depresses cellular-mediated responses. At higher and pharmacological concentrations the hormone has a number of inhibitory actions. Elevated estrogen, for instance, is associated with atrophy of the thymus gland. Androgens, by contrast, tend to suppress both humoral and cellular types of mechanisms.[11] An examination of the endocrinology literature reveals, however, that mechanisms through which sex hormones regulate immune and inflammatory responses are poorly understood.[12]

POSSIBLE ROLES OF ADRENAL ESTROGEN

I have developed an endocrine-immune blood test that measures cortisol, total estrogen, T3 and T4, and IgA, IgG, and IgM antibody levels. The measurement for estrogen includes all estrogen compounds in the body, that is estradiol, estrone, and estriol.

The test shows a consistent link between clinical signs of various illnesses and total estrogen outside of a normal range. Intact female animals are not tested during their estrus period. In out-of-estrus females, intact males, and neutered pets, normal levels are as follows:

- Males: 20-25 pg/ml
- Females: 30-35 pg/ml

Elevated estrogen appears to contribute to a number of negative effects:

- **Cortisol impairment.** Studies have shown that estrogen inhibits cortisol synthesis by specific interference

with enzyme activity,[13] thereby exacerbating a cortisol deficiency and initiating hormonal imbalances.

- **Thyroid hormone impairment.** Estrogen causes an increase in serum thyroxine-binding globulin, which may slow the entry of thyroxine into cells and thereby reduce thyroid hormone action in tissue.[14] Elevated estrogen may also directly inhibit thyroid glandular release.[15] Cortisol appears to be involved in the normal transference of T4 to T3, and the entry of T3 into cells.[16] By interfering with cortisol synthesis, estrogen may indirectly impair thyroid function. These combined effects may slow the overall metabolism and interfere with many basic physiologic functions.

- **Inflammation.** My patients' blood tests consistently show an association between inflammatory conditions and the pattern of low cortisol, high estrogen, and low antibody levels. Studies have shown that cortisol inhibits the production and accumulation of excess histamine in tissue[17] and the synthesis of prostaglandins, mediators of the inflammatory response.[18]

- **Cancer.** In humans, estrogens are involved in the development of breast and endometrial cancer.[19] All the dogs and cats I test and treat for cancer have impaired cortisol and high estrogen, along with deregulated immune cells.

- **Autoimmunity.** The same abnormal hormonal pattern is found in pets with autoimmune conditions. Immune cells are suppressed and appear to be stripped of normal regulation and the ability to distinguish between host tissue and foreign matter. Lahita has reported that recent data indicates "increased estrogen levels might initiate autoimmune diseases in many women and men."[20]

- **Aggressive behavior.** Many unpredictable and aggressive animals have the endocrine-immune disturbance. In humans, Finkelstein provides evidence suggesting "that estrogen may play a significant role in the production of aggressive behavior in both sexes."[21]

TREATMENT

I initiate corrective therapy when testing indicates the presence of imbalances. The protocol involves the use of various cortisone medications, either standard pharmaceutical compounds or a natural bio-identical preparation made from an ultra extract of soy. All plant material—the part of soy which increases body estrogen levels—has been removed. The compound is administered at low, physiologic dosages sufficient to compensate for deficient cortisol and re-regulate the immune system. These therapeutic dosages are significantly lower than standard pharmacologic levels used for short-term treatment and are usually needed for the duration of the patient's life.

This innovative use of a standard medication consistently restores lost immune competence. Most canine conditions require additional T4 thyroid medication. For some species-specific reason, most affected felines require only steroid replacement. This treatment approach has proven to be effective, safe, and free from side effects in thousands of cases.

After two weeks of therapy, patients are retested. There is usually a clear normalization of the key endocrine-immune markers along with parallel clinical improvements, indicating that a significant healing process is underway. In general, animals recover and maintain good health as long as the program is maintained. A supportive hypoallergenic diet eliminates the risk of food reactions which can nullify the therapy.

This clinical experience demonstrates the potent regulatory influences of cortisol and estrogen in immune function. It shows, perhaps for the first time, how an adrenal combination of abnormal cortisol and high estrogen interact to substantially deregulate and weaken immunity and contribute to multiple diseases.

For decades, William Jefferies, M.D., clinical professor emeritus at the University of Virginia School of Medicine, has used low-dosage steroid replacement for human patients with "adrenocortical deficiency" and reported improvement for allergies, autoimmune disorders, and chronic fatigue.[22] The medical community has largely ignored his clinical research because of an ingrained fear of using cortisone long-term under any circumstances. A similar fear exists in veterinary medicine. At conventional pharmacologic dosages, cortisone does indeed create side effects. In the past practitioners often shuddered at any suggestion of long-term cortisone, and, as the old saying goes, "threw the baby out with the bathwater."

Recently, resistance to long-term physiologic doses of cortisone appears to be eroding. Medical researchers have reported successful applications of low-dosage cortisone in rheumatoid arthritis,[23] polymyalgia rheumatica—a systemic inflammatory disorder of the aged[24]—and sepsis.[25] However, none of these studies link specific conditions to an overall mechanism wherein an abnormality of cortisol triggers excess estrogen, HPA destabilization, interference with thyroid, and deregulation of the immune system. I believe that this pattern of hormone-immune imbalance is a widespread but largely unrecognized mechanism among pets, and may contribute to various human illnesses.

TESTING THE HYPOTHESIS IN HUMANS

The presence of such imbalances in humans could most readily be tested among symptomatic men and postmenopausal (non-ERT) women. First, a baseline blood test would be taken to measure cortisol, total estrogen, T3/T4, and IgA, IgG, and IgM antibody levels, along with a 24-hour urine test for active hormones and other relevant markers. The urine test permits the clinician to compare results against the blood test. This is an important evaluation because some blood values (such as cortisol and thyroid) may appear normal in a blood test but in fact involve excessively bound, inactive hormone fractions. Blood tests alone may not indicate whether or not the hormone is working. The urine test helps answer this question and contributes to a more accurate assessment and effective treatment.

Jefferies' clinical experience with human patients suggests that low-dosage cortisol replacement therapy could be applied to symptomatic patients who are tested and found to have the endocrine-immune imbalances described in this article. If their health status improves and retesting shows a reduction in total estrogen, one could conclude that a hypocortisol syndrome with wide systemic impact has been clinically corrected. Such a result would argue for further investigation of this testing and therapy method for various illnesses.

Even though post-menopausal women are deficient in estradiol, their estriol and estrone are often very high not only from the possible interface layer but because the tissue enzyme aromatase converts DHEA and DHEAS and other androgens into total estrogen.

Gruber states that estrogen synthesis increases in non-ovarian tissues as a function of age and body weight even though little is known about the factors that regulate estrogen production in the post-menopausal population.[26] Longcope and colleagues observed a "marked increase in the ratio of estrogens to androgens in acute illness" among postmenopausal women. Conditions included heart attack, unstable angina, respiratory illnesses, and congestive heart failure.[27] One physician with whom I have been communicating commented that his sickest post-menopausal (non-ERT) patients have the highest total estrogen levels and the lowest immunoglobulins.[28]

Estradiol alone, and not total estrogen, is currently the standard measurement in patients, yet in postmenopausal women, estrone is the major estrogen.[29] Estriol, generally considered to be a weaker compound than estradiol and estrone, is present in significantly greater concentration in premenopausal women,[30] and may have significant though currently unidentified biological activity. I believe that total estrogen, including estrone and estriol, is a more meaningful indicator of estrogen activity than estradiol alone.

The presence of xenoestrogens and phytoestrogens, chemicals which mimic estrogen and which can potentially trigger androgen-estrogen imbalance, complicate the process of assessing serum estrogen status. Such compounds appear in the environment and in food. Ubiquitous estrogenic compounds, including industrial chemicals, pesticides, and surfactants, affect wildlife and laboratory animals' immune systems. Further studies are needed to determine the immune response in humans. These compounds may affect humans in similar ways.[31] Hence, the need to measure total estrogen.

Mesiano, demonstrated in 1999 that dietary phytoestrogen compounds found in soy decrease cortisol production and, as a result, increase androgens. Such consumption, he suggests, may indirectly increase total estrogen by raising DHEA and DHEAS levels. In his opinion it is "possible that some of the estrogenic actions of dietary phytoestrogens may be mediated via their stimulation of adrenal androgen synthesis."[32]

One way to determine the influence of dietary phytoestrogens, at least in men and postmenopausal women, would be to eliminate soy from the diet of patients who test high in total estrogen, then retest the patient again after several weeks. A clear drop in estrogen level could indicate a dietary effect. An unchanged or insignificantly changed level would indicate a source for estrogen unrelated to diet.

Xenoestrogens include birth control pills and chemicalized estrogen drugs. Can these contribute to a disturbance of cortisol and thyroid, and contribute to the disease process? It seems plausible that exogenous estrogen, or even androgen supplements (such as DHEA, which can convert to estrogen in the body) could indeed contribute to imbalances and disease.

My male patients' test results make a strong argument for hypocortisolism as a primary cause of elevated estrogen. In symptomatic males with endocrine-immune imbalances, high estrogen occurs almost exclusively as a consequence of a cortisol abnormality. The rare exception is the animal whose endocrine-immune status normalizes spontaneously without any treatment after moving to another area. I assume in such cases that a significant toxic or xenoestrogenic compound, perhaps ingested or inhaled, was present in one area and not in the other.

IMPLICATIONS FOR HUMANS

Elevated estrogen participates in a broad syndrome of hormonal-immune imbalances contributing to multiple diseases in animals. Is estrogen similarly involved in human conditions?

Is an unsuspected excess of estrogen involved in AIDS? Veterinarians regard diseased cats infected with feline immunodeficiency virus (FIV), a retrovirus similar to HIV, as untreatable. Yet I have a 70 percent recovery rate among symptomatic FIV patients. These animals have a typical pattern of low cortisol, high estrogen, and disturbed immune function. Low-dosage steroid therapy corrects the underlying imbalances and restores natural immunity. Cats remain disease-free as long as they are kept on the therapy. The results raise a number of questions.

Does the virus cause the disease or do the imbalances weaken the immune system and give the virus free rein? Do the imbalances also accelerate the disease process by deregulating the immune system so that immune cells attack both viruses and host tissue? Is it not possible that in humans cortisol-estrogen-immune status may dictate whether a person develops AIDS symptoms after being exposed to the HIV virus? My clinical experience with animals suggests that HIV-positive humans be tested for endocrine-immune imbalances. If present, appropriate hormone replacement might offer a significant prevention and therapy strategy.

All of my cancer patients have the same general pattern of endocrine-immune disturbance. Based on this experience I would suggest that human cancer patients be tested for similar imbalances. If they exist, appropriate hormone replacement therapy might offer an effective treatment strategy for humans just as it does for animals, even in advanced cases.

According to Gunin estrogen generates pro-inflammatory responses as well as proliferative changes associated with a pre-cancerous process in the uterus. Treatment with cortisone (dexamethasone) in ovariectomized rats given estradiol reverses these abnormalities.[33]

I routinely find the combination of abnormal cortisol and elevated estrogen in animals with histories of infertility and miscarriage, suggesting that reproductive failures may be caused by inflamed and immune-deregulated reproductive tract tissue. Such failures are routinely corrected by proper hormone therapy, enabling animals to conceive and produce healthy offspring. Over decades of clinical experience, William Jefferies, an emeritus clinical professor at the University of Virginia, has reported that patients with cortisol insufficiency and histories of ovarian dysfunction, infertility, and failed pregnancies achieve significantly improved conception and birth rates on low-dosage cortisone therapy.[34]

Common variable immunodeficiency (CVID) appears to be a grossly underdiagnosed enabling mechanism for a multiplicity of disorders in humans just as it is in animals, giving rise to chronic infections, autoimmune conditions, an increased risk of cancer, and poor response to immunization. In both humans and animals, CVID is characterized by low IgA, IgG, and IgM levels and abnormal T cell counts. In humans, the precise trigger for such immune dysfunction is unknown. Researchers have not linked CVID or other so-called immunodeficiency mechanisms to hormones. I suggest that exploring this connection, and looking specifically at cortisol activity, may generate major clues for diagnosis and treatment.

My clinical success and the growing clinical applications of low-dosage cortisone therapy for humans strongly argue for sustained research into the nature, magnitude, and impact of cortisol defects, including an associated estrogen-immune problem, in the etiology of disease. While it is now recognized that the hypothalamic-pituitary-adrenal axis, as part of the neuroendocrine system, has central importance to immune homeostasis,[35] we still don't understand the countless details and interactions.

Estrogen measurements are generally assumed to be expressions of ovarian function. This seems an invalid assumption, since a deficit of active cortisol—from genetics, stress, toxicity, or phytoestrogens—can initiate a significant estrogen buildup—estrogen dominance—independent of the ovaries. Estrogen dominance not only causes inflammation of many of the arteries, but it also binds active cortisol and active thyroid, and deregulates the immune system. It can also contribute to such ailments as cancer, autoimmunity, and hypersensitivity diseases. It will contribute to loss of homeostasis, deregulated immune function, and increased risk of disease among females with or without ovaries as well as neutered or intact males. In other words, none are exempt.

In humans, routine testing for a cortisol deficit and consequential hormonal-immune abnormalities, followed by an appropriate low-dosage, remedial steroid therapy program, may provide breakthrough strategies in the perpetual battle against disease.

REFERENCES

1. Munck A., Naray-Fejes-Toth. A. Glucocorticoid action. In: *Endocrinology*, Third edition, (Ed: DeGroot L). Philadelphia: W. B. Saunders Co, 1995: 1642-1654.

2. Ibid.

3. Parker, L. N. Adrenal androgens. In: *Endocrinology*, Third edition, (Ed: DeGroot L). Philadelphia: W. B. Saunders Co, 1995: 1836-47.

4. Adams, J. B. Control of secretion and the function of C19-delta 5-steroids of the human adrenal gland. *Molecular and Cellular Endocrinology*, 1985; 41: 1-17.

5. Alesci S., Koch C. A., Bornstein S. R., Pacak K. Adrenal androgens regulation and adrenopause. *Endocrine Regulations*, 2001; 35: 95-100.

6. Lemonick M. D. A Terrible Beauty: An obsessive focus on show-ring looks is crippling, sometimes fatally, America's purebred dogs. *Time*, December 12, 1994; 65.

7. Plechner A. J., Shannon M. Canine immune complex diseases. *Modern Veterinary Practice*, 1976: 917.

8. Harvey P.W. *The Adrenal in Toxicology: Target Organ and Modulator of Toxicity*, Bristol, PA: Taylor & Francis, 1996: 7.

9. Symington T. *Functional Pathology of the Human Adrenal Gland*, Edinburgh: E & S. Livingstone, 1969: 63-68.

10. Roberts E. The importance of being dehydroepiandosterone sulfate (in the blood of primates): A longer and healthier life? *Biochemical Pharmacology*, 1999; 57: 329-346.

11. Cutolo M., Seriolo B., Villaggio B., Pizzorni C., Craviotto C., Sulli A. Androgens and estrogens modulate the immune and inflammatory responses in rheumatoid arthritis. *Annals of the New York Academy of Sciences*, June 2002; 966: 131-142.

12. Cid, M., Schnaper H. W., Kleinman H. Estrogens and the vascular endothelium. *Annals of the New York Academy of Sciences*, June 2002; 966: 143-157.

13. Gell J.S., Oh J., Rainey W.E., Carr B.R. Effect of estradiol on DHEAS production in the human adrenocortical cell line, H295R. *Journal of the Society for the Gynecologic Investigation*, 1998; 5:144-148.

14. Arafah B.M. Increased need for thyroxine in women with hypothyroidism during estrogen therapy. *New England Journal of Medicine*, 2001; 344 (23): 1743-1749.

15. Gross H.A., Appleman M.D., Nicoloff J.T. Effect of biologically active steroids on thyroid function in man. *The Journal of Clinical Endocrinology and Metabolism*, 1971; 33: 242-248.

16. Jefferies W.McK. *Safe Uses of Cortisol*, Springfield: Charles C. Thomas Publisher, 1996: 160, 181.

17. Ibid, 106.

18. Orth D.N., Kovacs W.J. The adrenal cortex. In: *Williams Textbook of Endocrinology*, Ninth edition, (Eds: Wilson J.D., Foster D.W., Kronenberg H.M., Larsen P.R). Philadelphia: W. B. Saunders Co, 1998: 545.

19. Gruber C. J., Tschugguel W., Schneeberger C., Huber J.C. Production and actions of estrogens. *New England Journal of Medicine*, 2002; 346 (5): 340-352.

20. Lahita R.G. The connective tissue diseases and the overall influence of gender. *International Journal of Fertility and Menopausal Studies (now International Journal of Fertility and Women's Medicine)*, 1996; 41 (2): 156-165.

21. Finkelstein J., Susman E.J., Chinchilli V.M., et al. Estrogen or testosterone increases self-reported aggressive behaviors in hypogonadal adolescents. *The Journal of Clinical Endocrinology and Metabolism*, 1997; 82 (8): 2433-2438.

22. Jefferies, op. cit., 91-113, 163-166.

23. Hickling P, Jacoby R.K, Kirwan J.R. Joint destruction after glucocorticoids are withdrawn in early rheumatoid arthritis. *British Journal of Rheumatology*, 1998; 37: 930-936.

24. Cutolo M., Sulli A., Pizzorni C., et al. Cortisol, dehydroepiandrosterone sulfate, and androstenedione levels in patients with polymyalgia rheumatica during twelve months of glucocorticoid therapy. *Annals of the New York Academy of Sciences*, June 2002; 966: 91-96.

25. Klaitman V., Almog Y. Corticosteroids in sepsis: A new concept for an old drug. *The Israel Medical Association Journal*, 2003; 5 (1): 51-54.

26. Gruber, op. cit., 340-352.

27. Spratt D. I., Longcope C., Cox P.M., Bigos S.T., Wilbur-Welling C. Differential changes in serum concentrations of androgens and estrogens (in relation with cortisol) in postmenopausal women with acute illness. *The Journal of Clinical Endocrinology and Metabolism*, 1993; 76 (6): 1542-1547.

28. Personal communication with David Brownstein, M.D., West Bloomfield, Michigan.

29. Gruber, op cit., 340-352.

30. Wright J.V., Schliesman B., Robinson L. Comparative measurements of serum estriol, estradiol, and estrone in non-pregnant, premenopausal women: A preliminary investigation. *Alternative Medicine Review*, 1999; 4 (4): 266-270.

31. Ahmed S.A. The immune system as a potential target for environmental estrogens: a new emerging field. *Toxicology*, 2000; 7 (150): 191-206.

32. Mesiano S., Katz S. L., Lee J. Y., Jaffe R. B. Phytoestrogens alter adrenocortical function: genistein and daidzein suppress glucocorticoid and stimulate androgen production by cultured adrenal cortical cells. *The Journal of Clinical Endocrinology and Metabolism*, 1999; 84 (7): 2443-2448.

33. Gunin A.G., Sharov A.A. Proliferation, mitosis orientation, and morphogenetic changes in the uterus of mice following chronic treatment with both estrogen and glucocorticoid hormones. *The Journal of Endocrinology*, 2001; 169: 23-31.

34. Jefferies, op. cit., 67-90.

35. Cutolo M., Bulsma W. J., Lahita R.G., Masi A.T., Straub R. H., Bradlow H.L. Altered neuroendocrine immune (NEI) networks in rheumatology. *Annals of the New York Academy of Sciences*, June 2002; 966: xvii.

Importance of IgA

©Alfred J. Plechner, D.V.M.

Immunoglobulin A (IgA) has been a special interest to me as a major "yardstick" in assessing and treating endocrine-immune diseases. IgA is the most abundant antibody and is especially important in mucosal immunity. It is an essential protective factor against infectious agents, allergens, and foreign proteins which enter the body via the mouth, nose and upper respiratory tracts, the intestines, and the reproductive tract.[1]

In humans, IgA deficiency is recognized as the most frequent immunodeficiency.[2] Older studies suggest that up to two-thirds of individuals with IgA deficiency are healthy, but such conclusions are based on healthy blood donor subjects in whom deficiency has been determined from initial screening without any follow-up.[3] Recent studies indicate that as many as 80 percent of those who are IgA deficient but healthy may, over time, develop synopulmonary infections, allergies, autoimmune diseases, gastrointestinal diseases, especially celiac disease as well as gut and lymphoid malignancies.[4]

In animals, I routinely find low IgA blood levels associated with malabsorption and intestinal tract inflammation. This impairs the animal's ability to absorb both nutrients and medications. An IgA deficiency is seen in gingival buccal inflammation, glossitis, esophagitis, gastric enteritis, and food sensitivities.

IgA deficiency is also present in the following: respiratory system problems such as rhinitis, hay fever, pharyngitis, pneumonitis, and asthma; inflammatory problems of the kidneys, bladder, and urethra (often kidney and bladder stones are consequences of the imbalance); inflammatory reproductive tract disorders involving the uterus, ovaries, vagina (and frequently in early abortion cases); inflammatory joint disorders such as rheumatoid arthritis; and in patients who develop vaccine reactions.

It should be noted that these findings of IgA deficiency do not occur exclusively, that is, they typically appear as part of an overall pattern of humoral immune deficiency. I also test for IgM and IgG levels and finds that low IgA is usually accompanied with similarly low levels of IgG and IgM. It should also be noted that if in fact antibody readings are not all decreased there is a strong possibility of inaccurate lab results, since antibodies tend to rise or fall across the board, rather than in isolation.

CAUSES OF IGA DEFICIENCY

In my experience, compromised immunity—including IgA deficiency—among canines and felines stems from endocrine-immune destabilization originating with the zona fasciculata's inability to produce adequate cortisol.

Cortisol, a pivotal anti-inflammatory hormone, is the primary secretion of the adrenal glands in dogs and humans.[5] It also promotes the release of glucose to fuel the emergency response to danger and regulates the immune system. Normal cortisol activity is almost certainly required for proper immune response, according to leading glucocorticoid researchers.[6]

A cortisol deficiency in cats and dogs, which I first reported in 1976, appears to be largely a genetic defect[7] and quite likely exacerbated by current breeding practices.[8] I have found that deficient cortisol and IgA-related diseases occur through generations of families.

Other possible causes of cortisol deficiency include stress and toxicity, which may be significant acquired causes of cortical dysfunction. Harvey points out that the adrenal gland is the most vulnerable organ in the endocrine system for toxins, and within the adrenal gland the majority of effects occur in the cortex. Such disturbances can "fundamentally affect the whole body physiology and biochemistry."[9] Cortisol release is controlled by a classical feedback loop within the hypothalamic-pituitary-adrenal axis. The hormone is stimulated by hypothalamic corticotropic-releasing factor (CRF) and pituitary adrenocorticotropic hormone (ACTH). When blood concentrations rise to a certain level, cortisol inhibits CRF secretion. This then inhibits ACTH and cortisol secretion.

The androgens dehydroepiandrosterone (DHEA) and dehydroepiandrosterone sulfate (DHEAS) are the most abundant circulating hormones in the body. Known as prohormones because they metabolize into other hormones, these substances are primarily made in the zona reticularis strata of the adrenal cortex. They convert to androstenedione, androstenediol, testosterone, and further to the estrogen compounds estrone and estradiol.[10]

Androstenedione is the most important precursor of estrone, the most abundant circulating estrogen in post-menopausal women. Androstenediol, converted from DHEA, has inherent estrogenic activity.[11]

When the zona fasciculata cannot make enough cortisol, or for some reason the cortisol is excessively bound (inactive) and thus not recognized by the system, more ACTH is released by the pituitary to stimulate more cortisol. The zona reticularis also responds to ACTH. This tissue, as noted above, produces androgens that convert in some degree to estrogen compounds.

Excess estrogen promotes CRF release from the hypothalamus and more ACTH from the pituitary. This errant cycle appears to introduce a physiologically significant amount of extra estrogen into the system. Studies in humans show that estrogens inhibit cortisol synthesis by specific interference with enzyme activity.[12] If there is a cortisol deficiency to begin with, added estrogen would appear to exacerbate the deficiency and worsen the overall imbalance.

The term "estrogen dominance" has become popular in recent years. It is generally thought of as a symptom-inducing imbalance between estrogen and progesterone in women resulting from excess estrogen generated by ovarian activity, birth control pills, estrogen-like compounds in food, and other estrogen compounds in the environment. A problem of excess estrogen, originating with dysfunction in the adrenal cortex, has not been considered. In animals, I have repeatedly found elevated estrogen levels in female patients who are intact—though out of estrus—or spayed as well as intact or neutered males. The assumption is that the excess estrogen stems from adrenal precursors.

Hormone balance is regarded as a crucial factor in the regulation of immune and inflammatory responses. Generally estrogens in physiologic concentrations enhance humoral immune responses and depress cellular-mediated responses. At higher and pharmacological concentrations they have a number of inhibitory actions. Elevated estrogen, for instance, is associated with atrophy of the thymus gland. Androgens tend to suppress both humoral and cellular types of immune mechanisms.[13] However, the complex mechanisms through which sex hormones regulate immune and inflammatory responses are poorly understood.[14]

From a veterinary clinical experience based on testing and treating approximately 50,000 animals, low cortisol and elevated estrogen clearly exert negative, and often catastrophic, effects on the immune system. These effects consistently include lost disease protection as measured by reduced IgA, as well as low IgG, IgM, and T cell counts, and observable clinical signs of inflammation and disease. After so many cases, it has become abundantly clear to me that hormones in balance uphold immune system homeostasis, and hormonal imbalance destabilizes the system.

TESTING

I developed an endocrine-immune blood test which monitors cortisol; total estrogen; T3 and T4 thyroid hormone; and IgA, IgM, and IgG antibody counts. Comprehensive tests like these are not routinely utilized by either veterinarians or physicians. I initially included T cell counts in the protocol but dropped it because of the added cost to clients.

Cortisol itself, even if the value is normal, may be bound (inactive) to varying degrees in different patients. This is why it is essential to look at cortisol-estrogen-immunoglobulin relationships. The practitioner will recognize a cortisol problem if the estrogen level is high and the immunoglobulins are low.

Standard tests measure only one component of estrogen: estradiol. Total estrogen is a more accurate measurement since estrone levels can vary. Estrogens can exert a dramatic blocking effect on cortisol and thyroid hormones; just a slight variation out of the normal range is enough to cause hormonal and immune complications. In the presence of elevated estrogen, thyroid hormone may be bound or rendered inactive to varying degree, enough to slow down overall metabolism, and trigger additional problems. Thyroid activity may, in fact, be significantly compromised even if the thyroid values in the blood test appear normal.

The critical value of this test is that it offers a comparative view of endocrine-immune relationships. In this case, the relationships are usually low cortisol, high estrogen, and low immune cells. Retesting after two weeks, and periodically thereafter, provides a gauge for determining the efficacy of the therapy. If the immunoglobulin values increase, and symptoms decrease, the course of treatment is correct.

TREATMENT

Endocrine-immune imbalance is treated in a straightforward way. Cortisone preparations have many of the chemical actions of cortisol. They are, in fact, converted to cortisol in the body. The central modality I have used for thirty years is cortisol replacement with relatively low dosages of various cortisone preparations.

A second key modality, necessary in canine cases, is the parallel use of thyroid supplementation. (For some apparent species variation, only 10 percent of feline cases require thyroid.) Elevated estrogen has a binding effect on thyroid hormone. As a result, metabolic activity may become retarded, impairing detoxification and the liver's ability to process the cortisone medication. Thus, even low- dosage cortisone may accumulate in the body and, over time, create side effects. By giving cortisol and thyroid replacement simultaneously, at least in dogs, the patient is able to effectively utilize and process the former without side effects. Adjunctive thyroid should be considered in applying this approach to humans.

I consider 70-170 mg/dl the normal range for IgA in dogs and cats. Below 60 mg/dl suggests the presence of malabsorption wherein patients are unable to absorb oral cortisone. In such cases, animals are treated with IV (if they are critical) or IM cortisone. Malabsorption can be a significant factor even though there are no obvious clinical signs. Retesting after two weeks usually shows an increase in the IgA level. When IgA reaches 60 mg/dl, most animals are able to take oral medications. A small percentage requires continued IM treatment.

Correction of the disturbance with appropriate low-dosage cortisone (along with thyroid replacement in dogs) generally restores immunocompetence and health, even in critical cases. Animals deteriorate when therapy is stopped. Signs of previous illness return.

William Jefferies, emeritus clinical professor of internal medicine at the University of Virginia, has reported in great detail on the safe and effective use of long-term physiologic dosages of cortisone for a variety of human illnesses involving adrenocortical deficiency—allergies, autoimmune disorders, and chronic fatigue, to name but a few. This clinical perspective has been essentially ignored by the medical community because, as Jefferies notes, the "unique situation in which a normal hormone, one that is essential for life, has developed such a bad reputation that many physicians and patients are afraid to use it under any circumstances."[15]

Jefferies maintains that indefinite replacement with physiologic dosages of cortisone will benefit many, if not all, human patients with chronic allergies and autoimmune disorders, and that replacement should not be stopped upon initial remission.[16]

The treatment funds an adrenocortical deficit, corrects a hormonal derangement, resets the metabolism, and restores effectiveness to the immune system. Used therapeutically, it can save animals who might otherwise be destined for euthanasia. Used preventively to determine the presence of imbalance in asymptomatic animals, it can help avoid future suffering and premature death.

IS THIS APPROACH APPLICABLE TO HUMANS?

Does this endocrine-immune disturbance exist in humans? And if so, can a similar treatment protocol be applied?

The imbalance exists in every animal cancer case I have tested. Therapy outcomes are usually positive when combined with excision, chemotherapy, or radiation, even in advanced cases.

The feline immunodeficiency virus (FIV) involves a retrovirus similar to HIV. Veterinarians routinely euthanize symptomatic cats, yet I have a 70 percent recovery rate among such patients. They remain disease-free as long as they are maintained on low-dosage cortisone. Cats testing positive for the virus do not develop clinical signs once they go—and stay—on the program. Perhaps when a human is exposed to the HIV virus, whether or not he or she develops symptoms of AIDS may depend on the strength of their endocrine-immune connections. If an imbalance is found through testing, correction with appropriate hormone replacement could be a significant strategy for both prevention and therapy.

Can this imbalance contribute to human inflammatory bowel conditions? There is currently an epidemic of inflammatory gut conditions among dogs and cats. The imbalance, revealed by low IgA, is present in all affected animals tested. When the imbalance is corrected with therapy, IgA rises, absorption improves, and clinical signs resolve.

The same approach works for IgA-related conditions elsewhere. Animals with other chronic bowel disorders (including food allergies), respiratory and urinary tract disorders, and anaphylactic and vaccine reactions invariably have abnormal IgA levels, and improve after treatment.

I suggest that interested physicians test for the same range of hormonal-immune relationships in humans that I test for animals: cortisol, total estrogen, thyroid T3 and T4, and IgA, IgG, and IgM immunoglobulins. Other factors could be added, such as T cells and the androgen precursors of estrogen, in order to develop a more precise picture. Researchers have begun looking at the immune and inflammatory modulating effects of androgen/estrogen ratios and concentrations.[17]

Patients can be retested after biweekly or monthly intervals in the beginning to monitor changing relationships.

I believe there is a significant need to test for IgA in routine diagnostics, both human and veterinary, because of the importance of mucosal immunity for health. Currently, this is not done.

What is "Normal?" The Case for Standardizing Blood Level Scores

I requested several nationally known laboratories to provide the high and low levels against which they measured the blood samples physicians had provided. (See the chart below.) The wide variation in results seems inexplicable until one realizes that labs are largely responsible for determining "normal" ranges on their own—and often they base that determination on the last 200 to 300 blood tests run, rather than a set standard.

As a result, physicians tend to distrust lab results—and with good reason. Without a national standard defining "normal," it is problematic to determine if a score is abnormal. Standardizing "normal" levels among labs would allow physicians to evaluate readings more accurately and consistently.

I contacted eight leading medical laboratories in the United States. Following is a list of what each considered the "normal" IgA range.

"Normal" IgA Ranges at Leading Laboratories

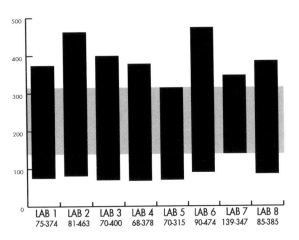

LAB 1	LAB 2	LAB 3	LAB 4	LAB 5	LAB 6	LAB 7	LAB 8
75-374	81-463	70-400	68-378	70-315	90-474	139-347	85-385

The discrepancies make meaningful comparisons, consultations, and discussion difficult among interested physicians. A patient may be healthy according to one laboratory's standard for normal, but unhealthy according to another's. Standardized CBC and blood chemistry levels are more or less accepted. Why is there not a similar standardization in major immune factors to help in diagnosis and treatment?

An additional factor to consider for female patients is the fluctuating nature of ovarian estrogen. The level of total estrogen will obviously vary according to monthly cycle, age, use of birth control pills, and/or estrogen replacements. One physician who uses hormones routinely in his practice was surprised to find that his sickest postmenopausal (non-ERT) patients had high estrogen levels and low antibody counts. A possible reason for this is the impact of low/bound cortisol and added estrogen from adrenal androgen conversion—a frequently overlooked source of estrogen. Estrogen synthesis is known to increase in non-ovarian tissues as a function of age and body weight.[18] Even postmenopausal women may actually be in a state of relative estrogen dominance.

Accurate test results among reproductive age women must account for and quantify ovarian estrogen's normal fluctuations throughout the menstrual cycle. This can be done by testing reproductive age females twice, once on the seventh day, when ovarian estrogen reaches its lowest level and again on the twenty-first day, when estrogen is highest. The difference between the two values will reflect endogenous and exogenous non-ovarian estrogen in the system.

The clinician might also want to obtain a 24-hour urine sample from the patient in order to test for active T3, T4, cortisol, total estrogen, and any other relevant markers. This would allow for a comparison to blood values, which may test normal but in fact involve significantly bound hormones. Without the urine test for comparison it can be difficult to determine if a hormone is available to the system or not.

Humans, like most canines, may require long-term thyroid replacement in addition to cortisone. Many humans have low thyroid despite normal values in blood tests. If thyroid function is low and the body's detoxification processes are operating sluggishly even physiologic dosages of cortisone could accumulate over time and generate the side effects typical of pharmacologic dosages. This was my initial experience in treating canines until adjunctive thyroid replacement was introduced.

CONCLUSION

I have not found comparable imbalances described in veterinary literature to match the scope of health-destroying suppression/destabilization of the immune system found in household pets created by deficient or bound cortisol and elevated estrogen.

In animals, genetics appears to play a major role. In humans, congenital adrenal hyperplasia (CAH) has some similarities. This condition is characterized by a deficiency of cortisol and an increase in androgens, the result of a deficiency in the adrenal enzymes that produce cortisol. Once considered a rare inherited disorder with severe manifestations, a mild form is said to be common although frequently undiagnosed. Patients with the mild form are often unable to mount sufficient stress responses to trauma and infection.[19]

It is possible that a similar enzyme disturbance could be operating in household pets? This may be the case, however, I have not tested for enzyme deficiencies nor for the androgen levels.

There are at least two clear dissimilarities. CAH involves hypertrophy of the adrenal glands and frequent deficiency of aldosterone, the mineralocorticoid produced by the outer layer of the cortex. No such situations are present in animals with the endocrine-immune imbalance.

One can speculate that a cortisol defect could be passed on to offspring if both parents are affected. In generations of animals an escalating severity of conditions related to this mechanism takes place. Might there be a parallel development among humans, with allergies and malabsorption in one generation and autoimmune diseases and cancer in the next?

Toxicity, as Harvey's work indicates, is another plausible explanation for adrenal malfunction.

Selye's famous work a half-century ago demonstrated that cortisol deficiency is a clear consequence of prolonged stress and contributes to some of the "diseases of civilization."[20]

Jefferies has examined the effects of mild cortisol deficiency due either to primary adrenal malfunction or secondary to inadequate stimulation by the pituitary or hypothalamus. He has reported that physiologic dosages of cortisone can improve a number of human disorders.

Recently, other medical researchers have reported successful applications of low-dosage cortisone in rheumatoid arthritis and polymyalgia rheumatica, a systematic inflammatory disorder of the aged.[21] CAH is treated, in part, with cortisone replacement.[22]

The veterinary clinical experience shows that a low-dosage cortisone approach is hugely beneficial and safe for restoring lost immune competence, including deficient IgA, and reversing clinical signs of disease. In this approach, testing for a serum IgA level, serves as a useful indicator at baseline of a hormonal disturbance to immune function, and specifically mucosal tissue immunity and inflammation. Once therapy has been initiated it again serves as an indicator of therapeutic progress. IgA counts are not generally conducted, however, it may be of great diagnostic and therapeutic value to do so. Open-minded veterinarians who have applied this testing and therapy approach have obtained excellent results. It has not been tested, however, in controlled studies. Nor has it been studied in humans. Such research is beyond the scope of clinicians, however, a controlled study on this testing and treatment method could produce major diagnostic and treatment breakthroughs for humans.

REFERENCES

1. Takahashi, I, Kiyono, H. Gut as the largest immunologic tissue. *Journal of Parenteral Enteral Nutrition,* 1999; 23: Suppl S7-12.

2. Primary immunodeficiency diseases. Report of an IUIS scientific group. *Clinical and Experimental Immunology,* 1999; 118 (supplement 1): 1-17.

3. Cunningham-Rundles, C. Disorders of the IgA system. In: Stiehm ER, ed. *Immunologic disorders in infants and children,* 4th ed. Philadelphia: WB Saunders, 1996:423–42.

4. Koskinen, S. Long-term follow-up of health in blood donors with primary selective IgA deficiency. *Journal of Clinical Immunology,* 1996; 16: 165–70.

5. Nelson, Don H., Samuels, L. T., A Method for the Determination of 17-Hydroxy Corticosteroids in Blood: 17-Hydroxy Corticosterone in the Peripheral Circulation. *The Journal of Clinical Endocrinology and Metabolism,* 1952, 12: 519-26.

6. Munck, A., Guyre, P. M. Glucocorticoid effects on immune responses. Unpublished paper.

7. Plechner, A. J., Shannon, M. Canine immune complex diseases. *Modern Veterinary Practice,* November 1976; 917. Plechner A. J. An effective veterinary model may offer therapeutic promise for human conditions: roles of cortisol and thyroid hormones. *Medical Hypotheses,* 2003, 60 (3): 309-14).

8. Lemonick, M. D. A Terrible Beauty: An obsessive focus on show-ring looks is crippling, sometimes fatally, America's purebred dogs. *Time,* December 12, 1994; 65.

9. Harvey, P. W. *The Adrenal in Toxicology: Target Organ and Modulator of Toxicity,* Bristol, PA (Taylor & Francis), 1996: 7.

10. Parker, L. N. Adrenal androgens. In *Endocrinology* (ed: DeGroot), Third Edition, Philadelphia: W. B. Saunders Co, 1995: 1836-47.

11. Adams, J. B. Control of secretion and the function of C19-delta 5-steroids of the human adrenal gland. *Molecular and Cellular Endocrinology* 1985, 41: 1-17.

12. Gell, J. S., et al. Effect of estradiol on DHEAS production in the human adrenocortical cell line, H295R. *Journal of the Society for Gynecologic Investigation,* 1998, 5: 144-48.

13. Cutolo, M., Seriolo, B., Villaggio, B., Pizzorni, C., Craviotto C, Sulli A. Androgens and estrogens modulate the immune and inflammatory responses in rheumatoid arthritis. *Annals of the New York Academy of Sciences,* June 2002, 966: 131-42.

14. Cid, M., Schnaper, H. W., Kleinman, H. Estrogens and the vascular endothelium. *Annals of the New York Academy of Sciences,* ., June 2002, 966: 143-57.

15. Jefferies, W. McK. Mild adrenocortical deficiency, chronic allergies, autoimmune disorders and the chronic fatigue syndrome: A continuation of the cortisone story. *Medical Hypotheses,* 1994; 42; 183-189.

16. Jefferies, ibid.

17. Cutolo, M., et al. Androgens and estrogens modulate the immune and inflammatory responses in rheumatoid arthritis. *Annals of the New York Academy of Sciences,* June 2002, 966: 131-142.

18. Gruber, C. J., et al. Production and actions of estrogens. *New England Journal of Medicine,* 2002, 346 (5): 340-52).

19. Deaton, M., et al. Congenital adrenal hyperplasia: Not really a zebra. *American Family Physician,* March 1, 1999: 1190.

20. Selye, H. Studies on adaptation. *Endocrinology,* 1937, 21; 169 (17).

21. Hickling. P., et al. Joint destruction after glucocorticoids are withdrawn in early rheumatoid arthritis. British Journal of Rheumatology, 1998; 37: 930-936. Cutolo M, et al. Cortisol, dehydroepiandrosterone sulfate, and androstenedione levels in patients with polymyalgia rheumatica during twelve months of glucocorticoid therapy. *Annals of the New York Academy of Sciences,* June 2002, 966: 91-96.

22. Deaton, M., et al, op. cit., 1190.

Reproductive Failure and Adrenal-Thyroid-Immune Dysfunction

©Alfred J. Plechner, D.V.M.

As a clinical veterinarian, I repeatedly resolve infertility and miscarriages in dogs and cats by correcting a common but overlooked hormonal-immune dysfunction originating with defective or deficient cortisol production. The key ingredient in the corrective program is a standard medicine used in a different way. This approach may offer insights into new ways of addressing reproductive problems in humans.

In the fifty plus years since they first appeared on the medical market, cortisone (steroid) compounds—the pharmaceutical derivatives of cortisol—have become prominent mainstream medicines because of their anti-inflammatory and immune suppression applications. Over the years we have also learned a great deal about the serious side effects cortisone may have when administered pharmacologically. Those side effects are the reason steroids are usually prescribed for the short term and avoided for prolonged use.

This development has discouraged interest in exploring cortisol's pivotal physiologic role in regulating the body's systems, the effects of cortisol deficiency, and the healing possibilities low physiologic doses of cortisone may offer. Cortisol deficiency tends to be off the radar screen of most practitioners even though the condition—which may result from genetics, acquired factors like toxicity or prolonged stress, or a combination of both—is common among both animals and humans. This is a major omission. Research indicates that immunity appears to be regulated by the hypothalamic-pituitary-adrenal axis,[1] and that normal health as well as reactions to stress and infections are critically dependent on the adrenal glands' ability to produce a proper quantity of cortisol.

In thousands of feline and canine cases, I have consistently identified a cortisol defect which sets off a domino effect of hormonal disturbance leading to immune deregulation. The result is an enabling mechanism for multiple disorders ranging from chronic allergies and viral diseases to autoimmunity and cancer. Special blood tests show that this pattern of disturbance

is present in animals—including horses who have been tested—with a history of infertility and miscarriages.

The signature pattern involves an initial deficiency of active cortisol plus elevated total estrogen, bound thyroid hormones, and low concentrations of immunoglobulins IgA, IgG, and IgM. This pattern is found in intact or neutered male and female animals. I believe that the elevated estrogen stems from a dysfunction in the hypothalamus-pituitary-adrenal feedback loop. The adrenal cortex, unable to produce adequate cortisol, causes prolonged release of pituitary ACTH. This in turn stimulates estrogen production in the adrenal cortex or adrenal androgen conversion to estrogen in peripheral tissue. The combination of low cortisol and elevated estrogen appears to interfere with thyroid function and destabilizes the immune system. Excess estrogen further binds cortisol.[2]

The medical literature contains considerable data linking thyroid function and reproduction. Indeed, many cases of infertility are treated with thyroid medication. However, thyroid hormones—both endogenous and as medication—may be rendered ineffective to some degree by abnormally low levels of cortisol and abnormally high levels of estrogen, which can bind the hormones, impairing cellular uptake, and interfering with T4/T3 transference. The metabolism slows, which can affect reproduction and even the body's ability to remove excess estrogen.

Low thyroid function in males is associated with impotence, loss of sperm production and motility, and abnormal morphology. I often see this in intact, though infertile, male dogs and cats with endocrine-immune imbalances.

Intact female dogs and cats with the same pattern of imbalances frequently develop endometriosis, cystic ovaries, and periods of excessive hemorrhaging, an apparent result of elevated estrogen. During a normal pregnancy period of sixty-two to sixty-five days such animals may miscarry. Sometimes gross fetal abnormalities develop—including small, mummified fetuses—followed by reabsorption. Could this be due to an estrogen-induced inflammation of the uterine lining? These female animals experience "silent heat," a condition in which estrus is not marked by typical vaginal engorgement or bleeding, and therefore often goes unremarked.

Blood tests of affected female animals often indicate normal levels of thyroid hormones but the action of these hormones appears to be bound, blocked, or otherwise hampered by elevated estrogen and low cortisol.

The hormonal disturbances compromise the immune system in general. Locally, the ability of the uterus to protect itself appears to be weakened. Blood tests consistently reveal low IgA levels, implying impaired immunity in the mucous membranes—including the uterus and ovaries—leaving them vulnerable to inflammation and infections and less able to host normal reproduction. In veterinary medicine, the cause of such pathology is frequently attributed to an infected male carrying brucella canis, a bacterium that can cause infertility and abortion. However, these microorganisms are usually not found.

As a prelude to corrective therapy for reproductive complications (and health disorders in general), I draw blood for an endocrine-immune test I developed. The test measures cortisol, total estrogen, T3 and T4, and IgA, IgG, and IgM levels. Because of wide and confusing discrepancies in the reference ranges of different laboratories, I developed my own range of normal values. Both males and females are tested. Females are tested out of estrus to avoid the influence of ovarian estrogen.

The correction process involves long-term, low-dosages of synthetic cortisone or a natural cortisol hormone replacement made from an ultra extract of soy or yams. All plant material—the portion of soy that contributes to estrogen dominance—has been removed. The exact type and amount of medication are determined by the weight and health status of the patient. During more than thirty years of practice, I have found that most dogs require cortisone/cortisol replacement along with a T4 medication such as Soloxine. Steroid replacement promotes transference of T4 to T3. When combined T3/T4 medication was used in dogs a suppression of TSH and reduction of natural T3 and T4 production occurred. Most cats require only cortisone/cortisol replacement. Horses generally require T4 alone, which appears to promote the adrenal gland production of cortisol and restore balance among key hormones and immune factors.

In this syndrome, cortisol and thyroid hormones are bound to varying degrees, and their individual values in a blood test may or may not appear normal. For this reason I compare the relationships of hormone and antibody levels rather than relying on isolated single values. The clear markers of imbalance are elevated estrogen and low IgA, IgG, and IgM. I retest patients after two weeks of therapy to determine if any modification of dosage is required. Decreased estrogen and increased antibodies indicate the effectiveness of this homeostatic "re-regulating" approach.

Correcting endocrine-immune imbalances in animals with reproduction complications has restored fertility and prevented subsequent miscarriage in more than 90 percent of my cases. However, both male and female breeding animals who are imbalanced need to be corrected.

Is a similar approach applicable to human reproductive failure? In humans, the use of low-dosage cortisol or cortisone medications to compensate for mild cortisol deficiency has been reported since the mid-1950s. William Jefferies, M.D., emeritus clinical professor at the University of Virginia Medical School, used this approach for patients with chronic fatigue, allergies, and autoimmune conditions, as well as for infertility and miscarriages where he found cortisol deficiency. In reports largely published more than thirty-five years ago, he cites consistent and significant improvement among patients, including improved conception and birth rates for many women with histories of ovarian dysfunction, infertility, and failed pregnancies.

Jefferies, now nearly ninety, has long and steadfastly championed the medical benefits of physiologic replacement of deficient cortisol, and lamented the fact that such use has been stymied by reports of cortisone side effects. Such side effects, he has repeatedly pointed out, occur only with large pharmacologic dosages of cortisone and do not develop with low-dosage physiologic levels when given to patients with adrenal insufficiency.[3]

"There is no evidence that patients who have taken physiologic dosages for over forty years have experienced any harmful effects, nor that children born to women taking physiologic dosages have any increased incidence of congenital defects or other difficulties," Jefferies maintains. My experience with animals bears this out.

Jefferies further notes that the treatment has an impressive preventive effect against postpartum depression and thyroid disorders. His findings about low-dosage cortisone therapy appear to be gaining wider acceptance today. Recently, medical researchers successfully used this approach for patients with rheumatoid arthritis[4] and polymyalgia rheumatica, a systemic inflammatory disorder of the aged.[5]

Many of Jefferies' observations about low-dosage cortisol replacement and reproduction parallel my veterinary experience. Such observations include:

- **Females who have difficulty conceiving also have a high incidence of miscarriages.** When low dosages of steroids are administered throughout the pregnancy to correct deficient steroid metabolism or a possible autoimmune disorder that interferes with conception, the incidence of miscarriage is no greater than it is among women who have no difficulty conceiving.

- **Excess estrogen can impair spermatogenesis.** The estrogen can be reduced with small dosages of steroids, which then improves sperm count.

- **Ovarian, adrenal and thyroid function may all need to be normalized before conception can occur.**

- **When properly administered, safe physiologic dosages of cortisol replacement (with thyroid medication, if necessary) seem to be an effective treatment option for ovarian dysfunction and infertility.**

Current treatment of fertility and miscarriage problems involves a variety of highly sophisticated and expensive methods. Exploring hormonal and immune imbalances caused by abnormal cortisol may yield new understanding and less expensive treatment options for reproductive failure, and should be comprehensively investigated.

REFERENCES

1. Cutolo, M., et al. Altered neuroendocrine immune (NEI) networks in rheumatology. *Annals of the New York Academy of Sciences,* June 2002, 966: xvii.

2. Plechner, A.J. An effective veterinary model may offer therapeutic promise for human conditions: roles of cortisol and thyroid hormones. *Medical Hypotheses,* 2003, 60 (3): 309-314.

3. Jefferies, W. McK. *Safe Uses of Cortisol.* Springfield, IL: Charles C. Thomas Publisher, Ltd., 1996:, 67-90.

4. Hickling, P., Jacoby, R.K., Kirwan, J.R. Joint destruction after glucocorticoids are withdrawn in early rheumatoid arthritis. *British Journal of Rheumatology,* 1998, 37: 930-936.

5. Cutolo, M., Sulli, A., Pizzorni, C., et al. 2002. Cortisol, dehydroepiandrosterone sulfate, and androstenedione levels in patients with polymyalgia rheumatica during twelve months of glucocorticoid therapy. *Annals of the New York Academy of Sciences,* June 2002, 966: 91-96.

Adrenal Toxicity and Hormonal and Immune Destabilization in Animals

©Alfred J. Plechner, D.V.M.
To be Published in *Journal of Toxicology*

Household pets are intimately exposed to a multitude of toxins. Among them are lawn and garden compounds, rat poison, insect and snake bites, anti-flea chemicals and other pesticides, antifungal drugs, anesthetic agents, cleaning and disinfectant solutions, lead in paint and water, building and decorating materials, synthetic carpet fumes, and a multitude of chemical additives contained in highly processed commercial diets. Sensitive animals may develop a variety of mild to severe symptoms following exposure. Immediate reactions include diarrhea, vomiting, ulcers, skin rashes, or anaphylactic shock.

In veterinary medicine, toxic overloads are viewed primarily as threats to the liver and kidneys, the organs of detoxification. High BUN or liver enzyme counts accompany actual toxicity problems. Once toxic exposure has ended and treatment has begun, one would expect the medical effects of toxins to be disappear in short order. In my experience, this is not always the case.

The adrenal glands are the most toxin-vulnerable organs in the endocrine system. The adrenal cortex, the portion of the adrenal gland where cortisol is produced, seems to be the most vulnerable to toxic damage. Such disturbances can "fundamentally affect the whole body physiology and biochemistry."[1] Indeed, the entire process of steroidogenesis "poses multiple molecular targets" for disruption.[2]

For more than thirty years I have focused my clinical practice on endocrine-immune imbalances, and specifically on a widespread but generally unrecognized defect originating in the adrenal cortex. The defect seriously affects cortisol production. In many thousands of feline and canine cases, I have linked a cortisol deficiency to a repetitive pattern of hormonal imbalances which compromises immune competence and acts as an underlying enabling mechanism for multiple disorders ranging from chronic allergies and viral diseases to autoimmunity and cancer.

In dogs and cats, this disturbance appears to be largely genetic, resulting from contemporary breeding practices. However, it can also be acquired in other ways, for instance, through stress, or through adrenal exposure to toxins. Whether genetic or acquired, the cortisol defect triggers systemic consequences.

Much is written about elevated cortisol as a normal reaction to stress and trauma, and about the anti-inflammatory and immunosuppressive effects of pharmacologic dosages of cortisone, the synthetic version of cortisol. However, at a basal level, the body's own cortisol exerts a discriminating regulatory effect on molecular mediators that affect immunity and inflammation. A normal level of cortisol appears necessary for a successful immune and inflammation response (see Fig. 1). Cortisol deficiency may result in an unresponsive immune system, while too much cortisol or too much cortisone medication suppresses immune responses.

In animals, I have found that a deficiency of active cortisol disturbs the hypothalamus-pituitary-adrenal feedback loop. As a result, pituitary adrenocorticotropic hormone (ACTH) attempts to elicit more cortisol from

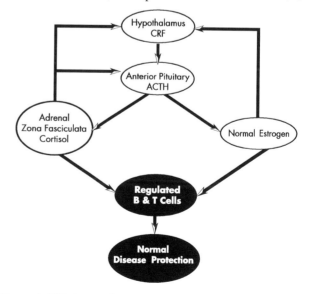

FIGURE 1: *This diagram shows normal relationships and feedback activity between the adrenal cortex and the hypothalamus and pituitary, and in turn, a healthy regulatory influence on the immune system.*

the cortical zona fasciculata layer. I have also found that this activity consistently promotes a measurable and physiologically significant increase in serum estrogen. The added estrogen may come from ACTH-stimulated zona reticularis androgens, some of which convert to estrogens in peripheral tissue,[3] or from "interface" cortical tissue that may directly produce estrogen compounds.[4, 5] In any case, consistently measuring elevated estrogen in all animals with the endocrine-immune disturbance—male and female, intact or neutered—demonstrates that estrogen dominance cannot simply be attributed to ovarian activity (see Fig. 2).

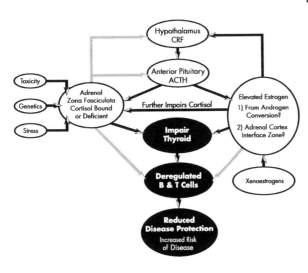

FIGURE 2. *Genetic and toxicity factors can interfere with cortisol production, triggering excess ACTH and estrogen release. Cortisol deficiency is aggravated, thyroid function affected, and the immune system destabilized.*

Elevated estrogen also appears to disturb the immune system.[6] In addition, the hormone also impairs the synthesis of cortisol.[7] Both cortisol insufficiency and elevated estrogen interfere with thyroid hormones.[8, 9, 10] I have observed that the combination disturbs thyroid function and slows down metabolic processes, including the ability to eliminate waste products. They remain in the body longer, undermining health. Toxins and medications that enter the body are also processed less efficiently, potentially leading to further harm and side effects. In short, this endocrine-immune disturbance renders animals less able to cope with stress, pathogens, and chemical and toxic challenges.

As noted earlier, toxins may also cause a cortisol defect. Such defects may be short term or permanent. My clinical observations over many years suggest that

the cortical zona fasciculata tissue, where cortisol is produced, is by far the most vulnerable adrenal target of toxicity rather than a more widespread cortical impact. A harmful effect on the production of aldosterone, synthesized in the zona glomerulosa, has been encountered only rarely.

TABLE 1: SERUM VALUES FOR DOGS AND CATS

CORTISOL UG/DL	TOTAL ESTROGEN PG/ML	T3 NG/DL	T4 UG/DL	IgA MG/DL	IgG MG/DL	IgM MG/DL
1.0- 2.5	30-35 female* 20-25 male	100- 200	2.0- 4.5	70- 170	1000- 2000	100- 200
*The range is for spayed and out-of-estrus animals.						

TABLE 1: *Normal endocrine-immune serum values for dogs and cats. Hormone values apply to dogs and cats of all ages. Antibody values apply to animals above the age of six months, or a month after their last round of puppy and kitten vaccinations. Antibody levels in younger animals may be suppressed, and not represent true values because of the impact of vaccines on immature immune systems.*

TESTING METHODOLOGY FOR ENDOCRINE-IMMUNE IMBALANCES

I developed a blood test which measures cortisol, total estrogen, T3/T4 levels, and IgA, IgG, and IgM, and serves as an accurate diagnostic tool for endocrine-immune imbalances (see Table 1). The typical imbalances seen in sick animals involve low or defective cortisol, elevated total estrogen, deficient or excessively bound thyroid hormones, and low IgA, IgG, and IgM levels. Years ago, a separate testing method to determine T cell function was conducted and showed that T cells were similarly weakened by hormonal imbalances. However, due to the expense of T cell testing this measurement was discontinued.

My endocrine-immune test measures total serum cortisol. But the number by itself does not really indicate whether the circulating cortisol is active, bound, or defective. The important question is whether cortisol works or not. The answer, I have found, comes from analyzing the other hormonal and antibody measurements. For instance, a low or even normal cortisol value along with elevated estrogen and low antibodies clearly indicates the presence of endocrine-immune imbalances. The cortisol may be excessively bound or defective. Either situation appears to promote elevated estrogen and contribute to deregulation of the immune system, expressed as low antibody levels.

Standard tests measure only one estrogen compound: estradiol. I test for total estrogen: estradiol, estrone, and estriol. This provides a more accurate indicator because any of the estrogen compounds may impair cortisol and thyroid hormones. In animals, a slight upward variation of total estrogen out of a normal range is associated with disturbed hormonal activity (for males, 20-25 pg/ml, and for spayed or non-estrus females, 30-35 pg/ml).

The test is based on a simple blood draw. After the draw at the veterinary clinic, the blood is spun down in a serum separator tube and refrigerated. It is shipped cold and refrigerated at the lab until testing. (If blood is not kept cold, results will be invalid, with artificially high hormone and antibody results.) Animals are retested two or three weeks after the start of therapy.

Imbalances are corrected with the long-term use of very low-dosage cortisone, which serves as a cortisol replacement. Depending on the individual case, either synthetic medications (Vetalog, Medrol, Prednisolone, or Prednisone or bio-identical "natural" hydrocortisone derived from an ultra extract of soy or yams is used. While soy plant materials can contribute to estrogen dominance, the extract, which has had all plant materials removed, has the opposite effect. Most dogs, but very few cats, also require a thyroid prescription (such as Soloxine, a T4 replacement) as part of the therapy program. This approach restores healthy antibody levels and effectively eliminates a major underlying cause of multiple diseases (see Fig. 3).

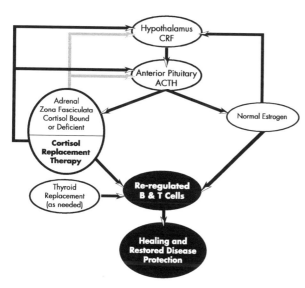

FIGURE 3: *Correction of cortisol deficit with cortisol replacement therapy restores normal hypothalamus-pituitary-adrenal relationships and immune system integrity. Thyroid replacement is typically required for canines, but not for felines.*

TABLE 2: ENDOCRINE-IMMUNE VALUES AT BASELINE AND AFTER COMMENCEMENT OF LONG-TERM TREATMENT

CASE 1	CORTISOL UG/DL	TOTAL ESTROGEN PG/ML	T3 NG/DL	T4 UG/DL	IgA MG/DL	IgG MG/DL	IgM MG/DL
BASELINE	.41	37.4	121	2.7	58	850	92
TREATMENT	.61	34.95	150	3.2	71	1200	130

TABLE 2: *Endocrine-immune values at baseline and after commencement of long-term treatment. Treatment values are based on blood draws usually conducted two or three weeks after initiation of therapy. Improved treatment values consistently parallel improvement in health of animals.*

CASE HISTORIES

■ Case #1: Permanent suppression of cortisol production

A three-year-old spayed female Old English Sheepdog presented with severe localized inflammation and swelling on the skin over the spine, the result of a black widow spider bite. A therapy program of antibiotics and anti-inflammatory medication proved successful.

However, a month after the conclusion of therapy, the dog started losing hair and breaking out in welts. She developed diarrhea and vomiting after eating her normal food. An endocrine-immune test revealed low cortisol, high estrogen, and low IgA, IgG, and IgM antibodies, a sign of deregulated B cell function (see Table 2). Previously, at the age of one year, the dog had been tested. Her endocrine-immune status was normal. Now apparently, the spider toxin had in some way damaged the cortisol synthesis pathway sufficiently enough to cause a deficiency.

The sixty-five pound dog was started on 40 milligrams hydrocortisone once daily and .6-milligrams Soloxine twice daily. Clinical signs quickly resolved. A subsequent endocrine-immune test yielded improved values. Note that the level of cortisol was still below the normal range. However, the dosage was deemed therapeutically effective. The combination of active exogenous and endogenous glucocorticoids brought the immune markers back to a level that re-established immunocompetence. At the present time, the dog has been maintained on the same corrective program for four years and has experienced no health problems. Periodic endocrine-immune testing has revealed normal immune values.

TABLE 3: ENDOCRINE-IMMUNE VALUES AT BASELINE AND AFTER COMMENCEMENT OF LONG-TERM TREATMENT

CASE 2	CORTISOL UG/DL	TOTAL ESTROGEN PG/ML	T3 NG/DL	T4 UG/DL	IgA MG/DL	IgG MG/DL	IgM MG/DL
BASELINE	.62	27.2	154	3.2	48	650	52
TREATMENT	.81	24.9	174	3.9	74	1100	121

■ Case #2: Suppression of cortisol following surgery

I have treated many animals who failed to heal properly or developed various clinical signs of illness after surgery. Testing for endocrine-immune function has routinely yielded a typical pattern of imbalances, suggesting toxic damage to cortisol synthesis from anesthetic compounds. When imbalances have been corrected with cortisol replacement (along with thyroid medication in dogs) the animals healed properly and their clinical signs abated.

One such case involved a neutered, eighty-pound German shepherd male. An endocrine-immune health check at three months of age showed no imbalances were present. At age three, the dog suffered a severe laceration on the left flank. At the animal emergency clinic, the dog received a standard pre-anesthesia (Keteset, acepromazine, and valium) and was then intubated for an inhalant anesthetic (Fluothane). The laceration was cleaned and sutured.

A month later the incision had not yet healed. The dog was brought to my clinic for evaluation. I performed another endocrine-immune test. It now showed substantive imbalances (see Table 3), which apparently affected the healing process. The thyroid values, although in the normal range, were interpreted as excessively bound due to the combination of low cortisol and elevated estrogen.

I instituted cortisol replacement therapy (60 milligrams of natural hydrocortisone daily), along with thyroid medication (.8 milligrams of Soloxine twice daily). The dog healed satisfactorily within two weeks, at which time he was retested and found to have significantly improved endocrine-immune test results. Even though the cortisol level was below normal it was apparently sufficient in this individual case to promote normalization and healing. The dog has been maintained on the same program for six years.

Case #3: Fatal dermal necrosis and suppression of cortisol

A two-year-old spayed female cat was being considered for adoption. The prospective pet owner wanted to be sure the cat was healthy and asked that I first test the animal's endocrine-immune status. The test revealed no abnormalities (see Table 4). The cat was adopted and joined another feline already in residence.

The new owner, concerned about the potential for fleas, purchased a popular anti-flea gel for her pets. The instructions advised direct application once a month to the skin between the shoulder blades. Shortly after the first application, the adopted cat developed dermal necrosis around the area of application. The second cat did not react.

The alarmed owner brought the affected cat to the clinic. Topical treatment with antibiotic and anti-inflammatory medication was initiated but failed to stop the spread of necrosis. I retested the cat for endocrine-immune status. The values were now significantly abnormal. The pesticide had apparently harmed cortisol synthesis.

A therapeutic program of low-dosage natural hydrocortisone (7.5 mg daily) was started for this ten-pound cat in order to correct the imbalances. Two weeks later, the cat was retested. The endocrine-immune values were now normal. However, necrosis continued to spread. Additional medical treatments were unsuccessful. The cat died ten weeks after having received a single—but fatal—application of anti-flea medicine. The cortisone therapy compensated for the cortisol damage but could not save the cat.

TABLE 4: ENDOCRINE-IMMUNE VALUES AT BASELINE, AFTER EXPOSURE TO PESTICIDE, AND AFTER COMMENCEMENT OF TREATMENT

CASE 3	CORTISOL UG/DL	TOTAL ESTROGEN PG/ML	T3 NG/DL	T4 UG/DL	IgA MG/DL	IgG MG/DL	IgM MG/DL
BASELINE	2.1	33.8	141	4.0	80	1500	160
AFTER PESTICIDE	.32	39.2	139	3.8	52	740	56
TREATMENT	.41	34.9	152	4.2	71	1300	107

TABLE 5: ENDOCRINE-IMMUNE VALUES AT BASELINE, AFTER RELOCATION ON CONTINUING THERAPY, AND AFTER DISCONTINUATION OF THERAPY

CASE 4	CORTISOL UG/DL	TOTAL ESTROGEN PG/ML	T3 NG/DL	T4 UG/DL	IGA MG/DL	IGG MG/DL	IGM MG/DL
BASELINE	.65	26.2	87	1.9	52	750	76
TESTING ON THERAPY, AFTER RELOCATION	.31	19.5	79	1.7	48	720	68
AFTER TREATMENT STOPPED	1.27	23.8	145	3.2	80	1200	140

Case #4: Temporary suppression of cortisol production

A one-year-old, seventy-pound, non-neutered male Doberman pinscher developed severe skin disease with multiple pustules. Testing for endocrine-immune imbalances revealed low cortisol, high estrogen, and low levels of thyroid, IgA, IgG, and IgM (see Table 5).

Imbalances were corrected with cortisol replacement medication (natural hydrocortisone, 50 milligrams daily) and a T4 supplement (Soloxine, .7 milligrams twice daily). The skin condition cleared up. However, faced with the prospect of maintaining the dog on a lifetime of medication, the owner opted to return the animal to the breeder, who lived 150 miles away.

Three weeks after relocation, the breeder reported that signs of cortisone side effects had developed: increased thirst, urination, appetite, and panting at night. I retested the animal. The results showed low estrogen and decreasing levels of antibodies, an indication of excess glucocorticoid presence in the body. The dog was weaned off medications and side effects vanished. A new blood test showed normalization of key endocrine-immune values.

The dog's previous home had been situated adjacent to a landfill and the confluence of busy freeways where unknown sources of environmental toxicity apparently suppressed adrenal function, resulting in imbalances and skin disease. The medication corrected the imbalances. Once relocated and no longer exposed to the toxins, the dog's adrenal function returned. In this changed situation, cortisol replacement medication had contributed to excess glucocorticoid concentrations in the body and was no longer needed.

IMPLICATIONS FOR HUMANS

The clinical cases cited above illustrate the extent to which various exogenous toxins may impact the zona fasciculata, suppress cortisol production, and create systemic disturbances. The endocrine-immune surveillance blood test I developed identifies a consistent pattern of hormonal and immune imbalances consequent to cortisol interference. A hormone replacement program based on low-dosage cortisone (and, in dogs, thyroid medication) has the potential to correct the disturbances and symptoms.

The endocrine-immune imbalances and medical effects I routinely see bear some resemblance to human immune deficiency syndromes, such as common variable immunodeficiency (CVID). CVID patients, for instance, have altered levels of IgA, IgG, IgM, and T cells, just as in animals. CVID patients also have an increased risk of cancer, particularly cancer of the lymph system, skin, and gastrointestinal tract. All of my cancer patients, with all types of cancer, have similar underlying endocrine-immune imbalances. Certain toxins may act as carcinogens. Does the route of carcinogenicity pass through the adrenal cortex and disrupt cortisol synthesis, which in turn causes additional hormonal dysfunction and destabilization of the immune system?

Researchers suggest that CVID likely develops from an interaction of genetic and environmental factors.[11,12] I suggest that studying cortisol activity may generate important clues for diagnosis and treatment of immunodeficiency conditions as well as cancer.

The chemical revolution has given us countless benefits, but it has also exposed us, as well as our pets, to an unprecedented volume of previously non-existent, potentially harmful compounds. We read continually of major toxic broadsides against wildlife that cause us to pause and wonder to what degree immunocompetence in humans is being affected. Recently, changes in immune cells, antibodies, and hormones among Arctic polar bears have caused concern among scientists.[13] The changes are a result of industrial chemicals called polychlorinated biphenyl compounds (PCBs) contaminating the marine food chain. Such chemicals can weaken the immune system with devastating results, such as when a distemper virus killed some 20,000 PCB-laden seals in Europe in 1988. Is it possible that toxic damage to cortisol synthesis contributes to such results? There have been a number of reports in recent years describing damage to adrenal cortex function in fish, including impairment of cortisol production, as a result of chronic exposure to heavy metals, pulp and paper effluents, and agricultural pesticides.[14, 15]

Defective or deficient cortisol is grossly underdiagnosed in veterinary medicine and appears to be so in human medicine as well.[16] A potentially major primer for disease may thus be off the radar screen of most medical practitioners. Moreover, many doctors fear long-term cortisone use at any dosage because of the drug's well-known side effects and its immunosuppressant properties. It should be noted, however, that such effects relate to pharmacologic, and not small, physiologic dosages of cortisone. William Jefferies, emeritus clinical professor of internal medicine at the University of Virginia, has reported for decades on the safe and effective therapeutic use of long-term physiologic cortisone dosages for human patients with adrenocortical deficiency. He describes significant improvement of allergies, autoimmune disorders, and chronic fatigue. I have also found that long-term, low-dosage cortisone therapy is safe and effective for animals suffering from these and many other conditions as long as the practitioner is correcting an underlying cortisol-based imbalance.

Jefferies believes that hormone replacement with physiologic dosages of cortisone should not be stopped upon initial remission. I find the same is true with animals. When medication is stopped, clinical signs return.

In recent years, successful application of low-dosage cortisone has been reported in rheumatoid arthritis,[17] polymyalgia rheumatica—a systemic inflammatory disorder of the aged[18]—and sepsis.[19] The benefits of long-term, low-dosage cortisone therapy thus appear to be gaining wider acceptance.

For humans, A test similar to the one I designed for animals could be developed to identify a cortisol deficiency in humans and assess health risks resulting from a genetic defect or environmental toxicity. Given the impact of hormones on the immune system, I strongly believe that such a test should become a standardized measurement of immune competency and be offered along with standard CBC and blood chemistry and other accepted diagnostics. If imbalances exist in humans as they do in animals, corrective treatment with appropriate low-dosage cortisone preparations should be considered as a remedial option. This therapy program represents a major healing modality for many seemingly unrelated chronic diseases of animals, including catastrophic diseases. In a time when the medical risks of environmental toxins are becoming increasingly worrisome, studies are warranted to investigate the validity of this type of comprehensive approach for humans.

REFERENCES

1. Harvey, P. W. 1996. *The Adrenal in Toxicology: Target Organ and Modulator of Toxicity.* Taylor and Francis, London: 7.

2. Harvey, P. W., Johnson, I. 2002. Approaches to the assessment of toxicity data with endpoints related to endocrine disruption. *Journal of Applied Toxicology,* 22,: 241-247.

3. Parker, L. N. 1995. Adrenal androgens. In *Endocrinology,* DeGroot L (ed), Third Edition. W.B. Saunders Co: 1836-47.

4. Symington, T. 1969. *Functional Pathology of the Human Adrenal Gland.* E & S Livingstone, Edinburgh: 66-68.

5. Roberts, E. 1999. The importance of being dehydroepiandrosterone sulfate. *Biochemical Pharmacology,* 57: 329-46.

6. Cutolo, M., Seriolo, B., Villaggio, B., Pizzorni, C., Craviotto, C., Sulli, A. 2002. Androgens and estrogens modulate the immune and inflammatory responses in rheumatoid arthritis. *Annals of the New York Academy of Sciences,* 966: 131-42.

7. Gell, J. S., Oh, J., Rainey, W. E., Carr, B.R. 1998. Effect of estradiol on DHEAS production in the human adrenocortical cell line, H295R. *Journal of the Society for Gynecologic Investigation,* 5: 144-48.

8. Arafah, B. M. 2001. Increased need for thyroxine in women with hypothyroidism during estrogen therapy. *New England Journal of Medicine,* 344 (23): 1743-49.

9. Gross, H. A., Appleman, M. D., Nicoloff, J. T. 1971. Effect of biologically active steroids on thyroid function in man. *The Journal of Clinical Endocrinology and Metabolism,* 33: 242-248.

10. Jefferies, W. McK. 1996. *Safe Uses of Cortisol.* Charles C. Thomas Publishers, Springfield, Illinois: 160.

11. Sicherer, S. H., Winkelstein, J. A. 1998. Primary immunodeficiency diseases in adults. *JAMA,* 179 (1): 58-61.

12. Lederman, H. M. 2000. The clinical presentations of primary immunodeficiency diseases. *Clinical Focus on Primary Immune Deficiencies,* 2 (1): 2.

13. Cone, M. April 2003. Bear Trouble. *Smithsonian:* 68-74.

14. Leblond, V. S., Hontela, A. 1999. Effects of in vitro exposures to cadmium, mercury, zinc, and 1-(2-chlorophenyl)-1-(4-chlorophenyl)-2,2-dichloroethane on steroidogenesis by dispersed interrenal cells of rainbow trout (Oncorhynchus mykiss). *Toxicology and Applied Pharmacology,* 157 (1): 16-22

15. Norris, D. O., Donahue, S., Dores, R. M., Lee, J. K., Maldonado, T. .A., Ruth T, Woodling J. D. 1999. Impaired adrenocortical response to stress by brown trout, Salmo trutta, living in metal-contaminated waters of the Eagle River, Colorado. *General and Comparative Endocrinology,* 113 (1):1 1-8

16. Jefferies, W. McK. 1994. Mild adrenocortical deficiency, chronic allergies, autoimmune disorders and the chronic fatigue syndrome: A continuation of the cortisone story. *Medical Hypotheses,* 42,: 183-189. 17 (Hickling et al, 1998)

18. Cutolo, M., Seriolo, B., Villaggio, B., Pizzorni, C., Craviotto, C., Sulli, A. 2002. Androgens and estrogens modulate the immune and inflammatory responses in rheumatoid arthritis. *Annals of the New York Academy of Sciences,* 966: 131-42.

19. Klaitman, V., Almog, Y. 2003. Corticosteroids in sepsis: A new concept for an old drug. *The Israel Medical Association Journal,* 5: 51-55.

Innovative Cancer Therapy that Saves Animals May Protect Humans as Well

©Alfred J. Plechner, D.V.M.

To be published in *Townsend Letter for Doctors & Patients,* 2004

Dogs develop cancer at about the same rate as humans. Cancer accounts for almost half of canine deaths over the age of ten years. Among felines the incidence is lower but a higher percentage of the tumors tend to be malignant.

Cancer has many causes. In my clinical practice I have identified a common, yet largely unrecognized endocrine-immune disturbance which acts as an enabling mechanism for multiple diseases, including cancer. I reported on this mechanism in the April 2003 issue of *Townsend Letter for Doctors & Patients.* (See "Unrecognized Adrenal-Immune Disturbance in Pets Offers Therapeutic Insights for Multiple Human Disorders" in this collection.) Over the last thirty years I have routinely tested thousands of cancer patients for endocrine-immune imbalances and found a similar pattern of disturbance in each and every case. The imbalances originate with defective, excessively bound, or otherwise deficient cortisol, an essential adrenal hormone with a key regulatory influence over immune and inflammation activity in the body.

The defect triggers a domino effect of physiologic disturbances, among them a profound destabilization of the immune system. The system loses its ability to prevent abnormally mutating weak cancer cells from growing rapidly. In one animal the proliferation of cells may develop into a skin tumor such as squamous cell in the jaw or mouth. In another animal, breast cancer, lymphoma, fibrous sarcoma, or leukemia may develop. The impact area varies from animal to animal. These are the same cancers that occur in people.

I have been able to resolve many cancer cases by addressing what I regard as a major causal factor—the cortisol defect. I have corrected imbalances in puppies from canine families in which cancer has already killed littermates. These "corrected" animals have gone on to live healthy lives for as long as they were maintained on a cortisol replacement program. Some did not develop cancer until eleven, twelve, or thirteen years of age. Some never developed cancer at all. Similarly, I have been able to save patients considered terminal. Even in these advanced cases, the cortisol replacement program I developed has often worked to extend the lives of otherwise doomed animals.

Cortisol-based endocrine-immune imbalances represent a major unsuspected cause of cancer in pets. I believe that such imbalances may be significantly involved in human cancer as well, and that exploring the cortisol's possible role may offer profound insights not only for veterinarians but for physicians who face the challenging task of helping cancer patients.

THE NATURE OF CORTISOL IMBALANCES

The typical endocrine-immune imbalances I see in patients, including those with cancer, involve low or defective cortisol, elevated total estrogen, impaired thyroid (T3/T4) function, and low IgA, IgG, and IgM levels.

Much is written about the dangers of elevated cortisol and the immunosuppressive effects of powerful

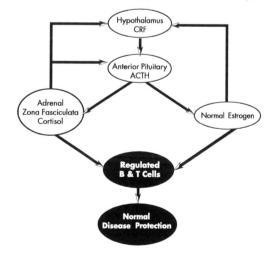

FIGURE 1: *This diagram shows normal relationships and feedback activity between the adrenal cortex and the hypothalamus and pituitary, and in turn, a healthy regulatory influence on the immune system.*

cortisone pharmaceuticals, the synthetic versions of cortisol. However, less appreciated is the fact that at a basal level the body's own cortisol exerts an important regulatory effect on the molecular mediators, which affect activity related to immunity and inflammation. A normal level of cortisol appears necessary for a normal immune and inflammatory response (see Fig. 1). Defective, bound, or deficient cortisol may result in an unresponsive immune system, whereas too much active cortisol or too much cortisone medication suppresses immune responses.

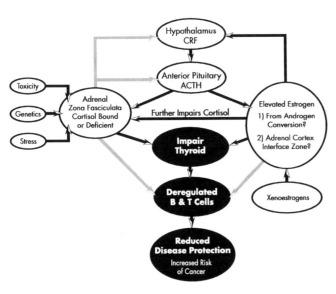

FIGURE 2: *Genetic and toxicity factors can interfere with cortisol production, triggering excess ACTH and estrogen release. Cortisol deficiency is aggravated, thyroid function affected, and the immune system destabilized.*

A shortage of active cortisol disturbs a primary hypothalamus-pituitary-adrenal feedback loop (see Fig. 2), and results in reduced disease protection, including protection against cancer. Adrenocorticotropic hormone (ACTH) from the pituitary attempts to stimulate more cortisol from the cortical zona fasciculata layer.

One consistent consequence of this activity that I have not seen reported elsewhere is the generation of a physiologically significant increase of estrogen compounds in the system. The added endogenous estrogen may come from ACTH-stimulated zona reticularis androgens, some of which convert to estrogens in peripheral tissue,[1] or from "interface" cortical tissue that may directly produce estrogen compounds.[2,3] I routinely measure elevated estrogen in all animals with the endocrine-immune disturbance—male and female, intact or neutered. Clearly, the excess cannot be attributed

to ovarian activity. It is possible, however, that environmental estrogenic compounds in industrial chemicals and in food (such as soybeans) contribute to increased estrogen as well.

Elevated estrogen disturbs the immune system in a number of ways, including interference with the thymus gland.[4] This interference has been implicated in the initiation of autoimmune processes.[5] Moreover, too much estrogen in the system may impair the synthesis of cortisol[6] as well as bind active cortisol, thus further exacerbating a cortisol abnormality. Researchers have discovered that phytoestrogens (estrogen compounds) in tofu and soy-based food decrease cortisol production and increase androgens, which can then convert in part to estrogen and raise the total estrogen level in the body.[7]

Medical science regards the hypothalamic-pituitary-adrenal axis, which is part of the neuroendocrine system, as a primary influence on immune function;[8] however many questions remain about its countless details and interactions. My clinical impression over the years has been that cortisol and estrogen have an intimate relationship which affects the homeostasis of the neuroendocrine system. If the relationship slips out of balance, the immune system becomes deregulated and disease protection is lost.

The combination of deficient cortisol and excess estrogen destabilizes the immune system and also appears to have considerable potential for interfering with thyroid function and slowing down the metabolic rate. Cortisol-estrogen imbalances can impact thyroid function by binding thyroid hormones, decreasing transference of T4 to T3, and impairing cellular uptake of T3. [9, 10, 11]

There appear to be several primary factors leading to a cortisol abnormality:

1. **Genetics** Breeding for cosmetic purposes rather than intelligence or function has caused a harmful narrowing of gene pools, which results in major health problems.

   Time magazine noted in a cover article that that there are more than 300 different genetic disorders that may subject animals to enormous pain and suffering. "The astonishing thing," the magazine article reports, "is that despite the scope of these diseases, veterinary researchers know next to nothing about what causes them or how to cure them."[12]

   The cortisol-based endocrine-immune disorder I have identified in pets may in large part be the result of these breeding practices. However, the disorder is not limited to purebreds; today these defects are widely established among all breeds—pure or mixed.

Many veterinarians are concerned about a sharp rise in cancer among younger animals. I now treat cancer in dogs and cats only one or two years old, something I never encountered when I started practicing veterinary medicine in 1966.

2. **Toxicity** Household pets are intimately exposed to many toxic compounds: lawn and garden compounds, rat poison, insect and snake bites, anti-flea chemicals and other pesticides, anesthetic agents, cleaning and disinfectant solutions, building and decorating materials, and a multitude of chemical additives contained in highly processed commercial diets. Sensitive animals may develop a variety of mild to severe symptoms immediately following exposure, but less appreciated is potential damage the adrenal glands, something I have seen in quite a few pets.

The adrenals are the most toxin-vulnerable organ in the endocrine system. The majority of toxic damage has been observed in the cortex, where steroidal hormones, including cortisol, are produced. Indeed, the entire process of adrenal steroidogenesis "poses multiple molecular targets" for disruption.[13] Such disturbances can fundamentally affect the whole body physiology and biochemistry.[14]

3. **Stress** Pets, like humans, experience stress. I have traced cases of imbalances in cats and dogs to household upheaval. Stresses may include owner divorce, transfer of ownership, constant harassment by children, the introduction of a new, incompatible animal into the house, boarding in kennels, and even too much exercise.

Mounting evidence in the field of stress research indicates that chronic stress can lead to a reduction of cortisol—not an increase as is widely believed. A persistent lack of cortisol may in fact be a frequent and widespread phenomenon, promoting a greater risk for immune-related disorders and other diseases.[15]

4. **Poor Nutrition** A poor quality diet fed over a long period of time contributes to systemic deficits, including lack of proper nutrition to endocrine organs producing hormones. Moreover, the complex nature of processed pet foods may not allow for adequate absorption of essential nutrients. Digestive enzyme deficiencies are commonplace, particularly in aging animals.

TABLE 1: NORMAL ENDOCRINE-IMMUNE SERUM VALUES FOR DOGS AND CATS						
CORTISOL UG/DL	TOTAL ESTROGEN PG/ML	T3 NG/DL	T4 UG/DL	IgA MG/DL	IgG MG/DL	IgM MG/DL
1.0-2.5	30-35 female* 20-25 male	100-200	2.0-4.5	70-170	1000-2000	100-200

*Spayed and out-of-estrus females.

TESTING AND TREATMENT

In 1972 I developed a special blood test to identify endocrine-immune imbalances in my patients. The specific measurements in the test are cortisol, total estrogen, T3/T4 levels, and IgA, IgG, and IgM. Table 1 shows my normal testing values.

Typical imbalances I find in animals with cancer and other illnesses involve low, bound, or defective cortisol, elevated total estrogen, deficient or excessively bound thyroid hormones, and low IgA, IgG, and IgM levels. Years ago I included a separate testing procedure to determine T cell function. Testing showed that T cells were similarly weakened by hormonal imbalances. However, due to the expense to clients of T cell testing this additional diagnostic procedure was discontinued.

In my analysis of test results, I place no great emphasis on the serum cortisol value by itself because it does not clearly indicate how much of the circulating cortisol is active, bound, or defective, and how much is actually working. I base my therapy decisions on assessing and comparing the other hormonal and antibody measurements in the test, which better indicate immune system function. Animals with a cortisol defect typically have elevated estrogen and low antibody test results, even if their cortisol reading is normal.

Standard tests usually measure only one estrogen compound: estradiol. However, I test for total estrogen including endogenous compounds (estradiol, estrone, and estriol) as well as estrogens from environmental and food sources. This provides a more accurate indicator than testing for estradiol alone, since estrogen compounds can impair cortisol and thyroid hormones just as estradiol can.

The endocrine-immune test is based on a simple blood draw. The blood is spun down in a serum separator tube, refrigerated, shipped cold and refrigerated at the lab until testing. If the blood is not kept cold, hormone and antibody results tend to be excessively and erroneously high. *Correct handling of the blood sample is critical. (See page 51.)*

Animals are retested two or three weeks after the start of therapy to determine the efficacy of the treatment and the need for modification. Imbalances are corrected with the long-term use of very low-dosage cortisone, which serves as a cortisol replacement. Depending on the individual case, either pharmaceutical cortisone medications or a bio-identical "natural" hydrocortisone derived from plants is used. Starting oral dosages are as follows: Medrol (methylprednisolone) or Prednisolone, 1 milligram per 10 pounds of body weight, or Vetalog (triamcinolone acetonide), .125 milligrams per 10 pounds; hydrocortisone, available through compounding pharmacies, ½ milligram daily per 1 pound of body weight.

Most dogs, but very few cats, also require a T4 thyroid prescription, such as Soloxine (levothyroxine sodium) at .10 milligrams per 10 pounds of body weight twice daily. Thyroid supplementation serves a dual purpose: to overcome any resistant thyroid impairment or binding effect due to endogenous cortisol-estrogen imbalances and to guarantee proper metabolizing/breakdown of the cortisol replacement medication within twenty-four hours. I have found that with dogs, but not with cats, even very low physiological dosages of steroid replacement have the potential to build up in the body and cause side effects unless T4 is taken as a daily accompaniment. For some species-specific variation, cats do not require the extra thyroid.

When animals are retested after therapy begins, the lab testing procedure cannot recognize the presence of synthetic cortisone medication as part of the serum cortisol circulating in the system. This is apparently due to the medication's different molecular structure. Thus, when synthetics are used, the cortisol value in blood tests will usually remain low. The test will, however, recognize natural hydrocortisone although changes in the cortisol value based on such usage may not appear immediately in test results.

The goal of therapy is restored regulation of the immune system. Even though the imbalances originate with a cortisol abnormality and the basis of treatment is correcting this abnormality, the most important indicator of efficacy is estrogen and antibody normalization, and improved clinical signs in the patient. In subsequent testing cortisol's re-regulating effect on the immune system is more important than the level of cortisol present in the blood. Again, I look at comparative hormone levels rather than empirical levels.

Special attention must be given to the IgA level. IgA is the most abundant antibody and is especially important in mucosal immunity. It is an essential protective factor against infectious agents, allergens and foreign proteins that enter the body via the mouth, nose and upper respiratory tracts, the intestines, and reproductive tract.[16] In humans, IgA deficiency is recognized as the most frequent immunodeficiency.[17]

Clinical experience has taught me that IgA levels well below 60 mg/dl reflect intestinal mucosa dysfunction, probable inflammation and malabsorption, including an inability to absorb medication. Low IgA is often the overlooked basis for inflammatory bowel disease. Animals with chronic bowel disorders (including food allergies), respiratory and urinary tract disorders, and anaphylactic and vaccine reactions invariably have abnormal IgA levels.

When IgA is moderately or substantially low I do not take a chance with oral medication, and certainly not for critical patients with an advanced, life-threatening disease. To ensure proper delivery of medication, I use intravenous drips or an intramuscular injection. My formula for IM injections is Vetalog (1 milligram per 10 pounds of body weight) in combination with Depomedrol (methylprednisolone, 1 milligram per 1 pound of body weight). In very critical cases I often double the quantity of both compounds. The former medication is an immediate-acting steroid, the latter a long-acting steroid that becomes active after five to seven days. Once the IgA level returns to near normal or normal, I switch patients to an oral steroid. Some patients who have had prolonged intestinal dysfunction because of low IgA may require monthly IM injections on a long-term basis.

CASE HISTORIES

1. Cat: spayed female, 10 years old, 9.5 pounds

In 1995, this beautiful gray domestic shorthair cat developed a large aggressive mammary carcinoma. Another veterinarian surgically removed the tumor but did not hold out much hope because of presumed metastasis. He gave the cat two weeks to live and suggested that follow-up chemotherapy would probably not make a difference.

The cat's owner came to me for a second opinion. I examined the animal and did an endocrine-immune test. The results from the test showed a typical pattern of imbalances (see Table 2).

TABLE 2: ENDOCRINE-IMMUNE VALUES BEFORE AND AFTER THE START OF ONGOING THERAPY.							
	CORTISOL UG/DL	TOTAL ESTROGEN PG/ML	T3 NG/DL	T4 UG/DL	IgA MG/DL	IgG MG/DL	IgM MG/DL
BASELINE	.41	37.0	123	2.24	46	840	72
THREE WEEKS INTO THERAPY	.33	35.9	140	2.28	56	980	94
FIVE WEEKS INTO THERAPY	.31	34.6	156	2.3	67	1100	106
ONE YEAR LATER (MALABSORPTION DIAGNOSIS)	.35	35.8	148	2.46	61	1050	98

The 46 mg/dl IgA level strongly suggested malabsorption. I initiated intramuscular therapy with a combination injection of 1 milligram Vetalog with 30 milligrams Depomedrol.

Three weeks later I rechecked the levels. The key values were improving. I administered another injection with the same potency as before.

After two weeks I rechecked the cat. The values had improved enough so that I could switch to oral medication—10 milligrams of Prednisone or Prednisolone daily. The cat was eating well and appeared much healthier.

In a follow-up visit a year later, it appeared that the cat might have some residual malabsorption from permanently scarred intestinal tissue resulting from years of low IgA in the gut. This may have caused a subclinical intestinal bowel disorder. A past history on the cat, other than the cancer diagnosis, was not available. I prescribed a monthly intramuscular injection of 2 milligrams Vetalog and 30 milligrams Depomedrol to bypass the gut.

The cat, now eighteen, has been maintained all these years on monthly steroid injections. The therapy was able to stretch a few weeks of expected survival time into many years of quality life. The owner still cannot believe it.

2. Dog: neutered male, 8 years old, 69 pounds

In June 2003, I treated a dying Siberian Husky. Two months earlier a previous veterinarian had diagnosed the dog with multiple metastatic lung tumors. The site of the primary cancer had not been identified. The patient was eating poorly, breathing with difficulty, and coughing persistently. The animal had lost twelve pounds since the original diagnosis.

I suggested doing an endocrine-immune test and proceeding immediately with steroid injections before the results came back. They agreed.

I injected the dog with 5 milligrams of Vetalog and 60 milligrams of Depomedrol. Test results showed that the animal indeed had endocrine-immune imbalances (see Table 3) including a 52 mg/dl IgA level suggesting probable malabsorption.

Two weeks later, the owners returned with a healthier dog. He had regained four pounds and was breathing easier. I rechecked the blood levels. The key estrogen and antibody levels had improved significantly, so I switched the dog to 6 milligrams of oral Medrol daily.

After another two weeks, I retested. The levels had normalized even further. Thoracic X-rays revealed that the lung lesions had disappeared. There was no evidence of tumors. The dog now weighed 78 pounds and had regained his appetite. Breathing was normal.

Although the dog has been on the therapy program for only a short period of time, the initial response has been excellent—and not unusual. The potential exists for normal health as long as the dog is maintained on the program. I suggested rechecking the dog every three months for the first year.

TABLE 3: ENDOCRINE-IMMUNE VALUES BEFORE AND AFTER THE START OF ONGOING THERAPY							
	CORTISOL UG/DL	TOTAL ESTROGEN PG/ML	T3 NG/DL	T4 UG/DL	IgA MG/DL	IgG MG/DL	IgM MG/DL
BASELINE	.68	25.57	114.6	2.59	52	914	93
TWO WEEKS INTO THERAPY	.60	25.01	130.2	3.2	67	1110	102
FOUR WEEKS INTO THERAPY	.58	24.67	129.8	3.02	73	1400	140

3. Canine parents and puppies

A breeder contacted me, concerned that her three-year-old breeding pair of Vizslas, or Hungarian pointers, had developed hemangiosarcomas of the spleen. Hemangiosarcomas are extremely malignant tumors that develop in the endothelium, the lining of blood vessels and the spleen. Death often occurs within a few months as a result of metastasis to the right atrium of the heart. Ultrasound determined that no metastases had taken place. In each case, the spleen was surgically removed.

I tested the dogs for endocrine-immune status. Both were imbalanced (see Table 4). As the table shows, the male was substantially deficient in IgA, indicating the need for an initial intramuscular steroid injection followed by a second injection after three weeks. I administered a combination of

TABLE 4: ENDOCRINE-IMMUNE VALUES BEFORE AND AFTER THE START OF ONGOING THERAPY

MALE VIZSLA	CORTISOL UG/DL	TOTAL ESTROGEN PG/ML	T3 NG/DL	T4 UG/DL	IGA MG/DL	IGG MG/DL	IGM MG/DL
BASELINE	.32	27.25	99.2	1.98	43	796	68
SIX WEEKS INTO THERAPY	.29	24.9	118	2.76	60	1030	108
AT EIGHT WEEKS	.30	23.4	130	3.1	76	1390	152
FEMALE VIZSLA							
BASELINE	.49	38.1	112	2.1	41	690	65
SIX WEEKS INTO THERAPY	.46	36.01	137	2.37	58	900	86
EIGHT WEEKS	.40	35.01	151	2.61	70	1100	106

5 milligrams Vetalog with 60 milligrams Depomedrol to the sixty-five-pound dog and prescribed .6 milligrams of Soloxine twice daily orally. (The relatively small molecular structure of T4 medication is more easily absorbed than compounds such as steroids with their larger molecular size).

At six weeks the dog was retested. The levels had improved considerably. I switched the animal to 6 milligrams daily of oral Medrol. Retesting after another two weeks showed further normalization.

The fifty-two pound female was examined, tested, and treated at the same time as the male. Her endocrine-immune levels were similarly abnormal. I injected her twice over a three-week period with 4 milligrams of Vetalog and 50 milligrams of Depomedrol, and prescribed .5 milligrams of T4 replacement twice daily. When her values normalized, I switched her to 4 milligrams of oral Medrol.

Both dogs have been maintained on this program since that time, are in good health, and happily involved in hunting activities.

When parents have similar imbalances, as these dogs did, experience has shown that the offspring will likely have the same abnormalities and are at high risk of developing the same cancer.

The male and female Vizslas had produced a litter of six puppies about one year before their operation. Shortly after treating the parents these one-year-old puppies—four males (54-60 pounds) and two females (50-56 pounds)—were tested for endocrine-immune imbalances (see Table 5).

The puppies each had a similar pattern of endocrine-immune imbalances. The breeder agreed that the best preventive strategy was to normalize these imbalances with a proper hormone replacement program. The young dogs were placed on a combination of steroids

(Medrol) and T4 medication, with dosages calculated according to their individual weight.

Four years later, the puppies and parents are still maintained on the program. No cancer has occurred during this time. Blood tests performed by other veterinarians in other parts of the country are normal. The dogs remain on the program.

DISCUSSION AND IMPLICATIONS FOR HUMANS

The testing and therapy program described here has produced outstanding results for many years. I have used it successfully to identify and correct a causal adrenal defect that weakens and destabilizes the immune system as well as to treat many different types of cancer.

The program can improve both length and quality of life for animal cancer patients if their physical condition has not been severely compromised by the disease. The earlier in the disease process that treatment begins the greater the potential for containment and recovery. The program will often prevent cancer from recurring or spreading.

Correcting the endocrine-immune defect restores impaired functions and often prevents cancer in genetically predisposed animals, and keeps the disease in check for many years in cases where it occurs.

Surgery, radiation, and chemotherapy are often indicated to eliminate tumors. The hormone replacement program is highly supportive, and, in fact, may ensure the success of those treatments. Conventional methods may not stop recurrence, but in conjunction with the replacement therapy there may be total containment. Whether the cancer is advanced or still in

TABLE 5: ENDOCRINE-IMMUNE VALUES BEFORE START OF ONGOING THERAPY AND TWO WEEKS INTO PROGRAM.

	CORTISOL UG/DL	TOTAL ESTROGEN PG/ML	T3 NG/DL	T4 UG/DL	IGA MG/DL	IGG MG/DL	IGM MG/DL
MALE #1 BASELINE	.30	25.9	110	2.1	58	980	88
THERAPY, 2 WKS	.32	24.1	116	2.43	78	1290	118.6
MALE #2	.37	26.0	114	2.3	54	890	83
THERAPY, 2 WKS	.39	25.01	121	2.51	76	1180	110.2
MALE #3	.35	25.6	108	2.51	61	990	85
THERAPY, 2 WKS	.34	24.6	111	2.67	77	1325	112.3
MALE #4	.38	25.8	112	2.4	59	910	81
THERAPY, 2 WKS	.40	23.9	119	2.90	89	1465	131.1
FEMALE #1	.31	36.7	120	2.27	56	870	78
THERAPY, 2 WKS	.33	34.8	122	2.44	74	1275	111.8
FEMALE #2	.34	36.2	118	2.16	64	880	92
THERAPY, 2 WKS	.36	34.6	121	2.39	77	1340	116

its early stages, repairing the defective endocrine-immune mechanism restores the patient's own powerful self-healing potential. Without this basic repair work, healing may never take place.

William Jefferies, M.D., retired endocrinologist and professor emeritus of internal medicine at the University of Virginia, has reported for decades on the safe and effective therapeutic use of long-term physiologic dosages of cortisone in human patients with adrenocortical deficiency. He describes significant alleviation of allergies, autoimmune disorders, and chronic fatigue, and further suggests the potential benefits of low-dosage approach as part of a comprehensive cancer treatment program. In his book, *Safe Uses of Cortisol,* Jefferies notes that the persistent application of physiologic dosages of appropriate steroids "might help patients with any type of malignancy by improving their resistance to cancer."[18] Defective, bound, or deficient cortisol is grossly underdiagnosed in veterinary medicine and appears to be so in human medicine as well.[19] Many doctors, moreover, still fear long-term cortisone use at any dosage because of the drug's well-known side effects and its immunosuppressant properties. It should be noted, however, that such effects relate to comparatively large pharmacologic dosages, not small physiologic dosages. As I have found, Jefferies maintains that replacement with physiologic dosages of cortisone should not be stopped upon initial remission. When medication is stopped, clinical signs return.

In recent years, successful application of low-dosage cortisone has been reported in rheumatoid arthritis,[20] polymyalgia rheumatica—a systemic inflammatory disorder of the aged[21]—and sepsis.[22] The benefits of long-term, low-dosage cortisone therapy thus appears to be gaining wider acceptance, perhaps due to a better understanding of cortisol's vital role in immune regulation.

Do my findings in animals with cancer apply to humans? Can cortisol deficiency, for whatever reason, increase the risk of cancer?

Congenital adrenal hyperplasia (CAH) is a human disease in which the enzymes involved in the synthesis of cortisol are impaired, resulting in a cortisol deficiency. Unless treated with steroids, patients cannot mount sufficient response to stress and infections. Researchers have found a significant prevalence of testicular cancer among CAH patients.[23]

The endocrine-immune imbalances and medical effects I routinely see bear some resemblance to human immune deficiency syndromes, notably common variable immunodeficiency (CVID). CVID patients have deficient levels of IgA, IgG, IgM and T cells, just like the sick animals I treat. Interestingly, CVID patients also have the same predisposition to chronic infections, autoimmune conditions, and intestinal bowel disease, as well as an increased risk of cancer, particularly cancer of the lymph system, skin, and gastrointestinal tract. Experts say that CVID is probably caused by an interaction of genetic and acquired factors.[24, 25]

For more than thirty years I have observed generations of animals and witnessed an escalating severity of conditions related to cortisol problems. It wouldn't surprise me to learn that there is a parallel development among humans: allergies and malabsorption in one generation and autoimmune diseases and cancer in the next.

As I have noted earlier, toxicity affects the adrenal cortex more than any other organ within the endocrine system. Some toxins may act as carcinogens. Thus a main route of carcinogenicity may pass through the adrenal cortex and disrupt cortisol synthesis, which in turn causes additional hormonal dysfunction and immune system destabilization.

The chemical revolution has given us countless benefits, but at the same time has exposed us to an unprecedented volume of previously non-existent potentially harmful compounds. We read continually of toxic broadsides against wildlife that leave us wondering to what degree immunocompetence in humans is being affected. Recently, changes in immune cells, antibodies, and hormones among Arctic polar bears have caused concern among scientists.[26] The changes are a result of industrial chemicals called polychlorinated biphenyl compounds (PCBs) contaminating the marine food chain. Such chemicals can weaken the immune system with devastating results. A distemper virus killed some 20,000 PCB-laden seals in Europe in 1988. Is it possible that toxic damage to cortisol synthesis contributes to such end results? There have been a number of reports in recent years describing damage to adrenal cortex function in fish, including impairment of cortisol production as a result of chronic exposure to heavy metals, pulp and paper effluents, and agricultural pesticides.[27, 28]

A growing body of research indicates that chronic stress depletes cortisol and increases vulnerability for stress-related physical disorders. According to the National Cancer Institute, however, no direct relationship between psychological stress and cancer occurrence or progression has been scientifically proven.[29]

Elevated estrogen's role in the endocrine-immune syndrome I have described deserves special attention. In humans, estrogens are involved in the development of breast and endometrial cancer.[30]

Estrogen measurements are generally assumed to be expressions of ovarian function. However, this is obviously an invalid assumption, given the exposure to estrogens in environmental chemicals and food, birth control pills, estrogen replacement therapy, and the added factor of adrenally-induced estrogen. I have found no reports in the medical literature of estrogen elevated as a result of the active cortisol deficit I have found and reported in animals. From my viewpoint, this overlooked element of added estrogen clearly contributes to a situation popularly referred to as "estrogen dominance," which may lead to a loss of homeostasis, reduced immune function, and increased risk of catastrophic disease.

A Russian study on uterine tissue in ovariectomized rats who received estrogen (estradiol). The rats developed pro-inflammatory responses and proliferative changes associated with a pre-cancerous process. Treatment with cortisone (dexamethasone) reversed these abnormalities.[31]

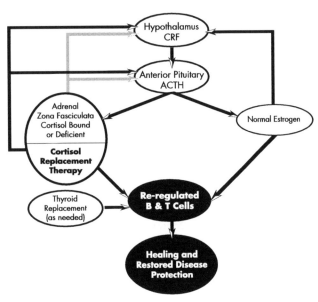

FIGURE 3: *Correction of cortisol deficit with cortisol replacement therapy restores normal hypothalamus-pituitary-adrenal relationships and immune system integrity. Thyroid replacement is typically required for canines, but not for felines.*

CONCLUSIONS

Based on my clinical experience and that of other veterinarians who use my testing and treatment method, the cortisol-cancer connection certainly seems to warrant investigation in the field of human medicine.

Testing must include IgA because of the importance of mucosal immunity for health proper absorption. If malabsorption exists, medication may not reach the systems it needs to affect. Currently, IgA is not included in general diagnostics.

In this context, there is a need to standardize testing procedures and reference ranges for such testing. Following is a list of "normal" IgA ranges at eight leading medical laboratories in the United States.

"NORMAL" IGA RANGES AT LEADING LABORATORIES

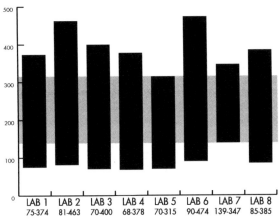

Such discrepancies make it difficult for comparisons, consultations and discussion among interested physicians. A patient could be "healthy" according to one laboratory's standard, but unhealthy according to another's. Standardized CBC and blood chemistry levels are more or less accepted. There should be major immune factor scores standardization as well to help us in the diagnosis and treatment of critically-ill patients. IgA is just one factor, but a big one, since it must be monitored at baseline. If IgA is low, there may be a problem with malabsorption. Retest after two or three weeks of therapy. If there is no improvement in testing values or in clinical signs then malabsorption is likely present and treatment then requires an intramuscular injection as I describe.

The Endocrine-Immune (E-I) panel I developed and successfully use for animals is increasingly being used by physicians to evaluate their human patients. Routine testing for a cortisol deficit and its hormonal and immune system consequences may provide breakthrough diagnostic clues for humans just as they have in my animal practice. If such abnormalities exist, treatment with sustained low-dosage steroids and possibly thyroid supplementation as well may offer a powerful strategy in the battle against cancer.

REFERENCES

1. Parker, L. N. Adrenal androgens. In: *Endocrinology*, Third edition, (Ed: DeGroot, L). Philadelphia: W. B. Saunders Co, 1995: 1836-47.

2. Symington, T. *Functional Pathology of the Human Adrenal Gland.* Edinburgh: E & S Livingstone, 1969: 66-68.

3. Roberts, E. The importance of being dehydroepiandrosterone sulfate. *Biochemical Pharmacology*, 1999; 57: 329-46.

4. Cutolo, M., Seriolo, B., Villaggio, B., Pizzorni, C., Craviotto, C., Sulli, A. Androgens and estrogens modulate the immune and inflammatory responses in rheumatoid arthritis. *Annals of the New York Academy of Sciences*, June 2002; 966: 131-42.

5. Lahita, R. The connective tissue diseases and the overall influence of gender. *International Journal of Fertility and Menopausal Studies (Now International Journal of Fertility and Women's Medicine)*, 1996; 41 (2):156-165.

6. Gell, J.S., Oh, J., Rainey, W.E., Carr, B.R. Effect of estradiol on DHEAS production in the human adrenocortical cell line, H295R. *Journal of the Society for Gynecologic Investigation*, 1998; 5: 144-48.

7. Mesiano, S., Katz, S. L., Lee, J. Y., Jaffe, R. B. Phytoestrogens alter adrenocortical function: genistein and daidzein suppress glucocorticoid and stimulate androgen production by cultured adrenal cortical cells. *The Journal of Clinical Endocrinology and Metabolism*, 1999; 84 (7): 2443-2448.

8. Cutolo, M., et al. Altered neuroendocrine immune (NEI) networks in rheumatology. *Annals of the New York Academy of Sciences*, June 2002; 966: xvii.

9. Arafah, B. M. Increased need for thyroxine in women with hypothyroidism during estrogen therapy. *New England Journal of Medicine*, 2001; 344 (23): 1743-1749.

10. Gross, H. A., Appleman, M. D., Nicoloff, J. T. Effect of biologically active steroids on thyroid function in man. *The Journal of Clinical Endocrinology and Metabolism*, 1971; 33: 242-248.

11. Jefferies, W. McK. *Safe Uses of Cortisol.* Springfield: Charles C. Thomas Publisher, 1996: 160, 181.

12. Lemonick, M. D. A Terrible Beauty: An obsessive focus on show-ring looks is crippling, sometimes fatally, America's purebred dogs. *Time*, December 12, 1994; 65.

13. Harvey, P. W., Johnson, I. Approaches to the assessment of toxicity data with endpoints related to endocrine disruption. *Journal of Applied Toxicology*, 2002; 22: 241-247.

14. Harvey, P. W. The Adrenal in *Toxicology: Target Organ and Modulator of Toxicity.* Bristol, PA: Taylor & Francis, 1996: 7.

15. Heim, C., Ehlert, U., Hellhammer, D. H. The potential role of hypocortisolism in the pathophysiology of stress-related bodily disorders. *Psychoneuroendocrinology*, 2000; 25: 1-35.

16. Takahashi, I., Kiyono, H. Gut as the largest immunologic tissue. *Journal of Parenteral Enteral Nutrition*, 1999; 23: Suppl S7-12.

17. Primary immunodeficiency diseases. Report of an International Union of Immunological Societies scientific group. *Clinical and Experimental Immunology*, 1999; 118 (supplement 1): 1-17.

18. Jefferiesm, W. McK. Op. cit., 165.

19. Jefferies, W. McK. Mild adrenocortical deficiency, chronic allergies, autoimmune disorders and the chronic fatigue syndrome: A continuation of the cortisone story. *Medical Hypotheses*, 1994; 42: 183-189.

20. Hickling, P., Jacoby, R. K., Kirwan, J. R. Joint destruction after glucocorticoids are withdrawn in early rheumatoid arthritis. *British Journal of Rheumatology*, 1998; 37: 930-936.

21. Cutolo, M., Sulli, A., Pizzorni, C., et al. Cortisol, dehydroepiandrosterone sulfate, and androstenedione levels in patients with polymyalgia rheumatica during twelve months of glucocorticoid therapy. *Annals of the New York Academy of Sciences*, June 2002; 966: 91-96.

22. Klaitman, V., Almog, Y. Corticosteroids in sepsis: A new concept for an old drug. *The Israel Medical Association Journal*, 2003; 5 (1): 51-54.

23. Stickkelbroeck, N. M., Otten, B. J., Pasic, A., et al. High prevalence of testicular adrenal rest tumors, impaired spermatogenesis, and Leydig cell failure in adolescent and adult males with congenital adrenal hyperplasia. *The Journal of Clinical Endocrinology and Metabolism*, 2001; 86 (12): 5721-5728.

24. Sicherer, S. H., Winkelstein, J. A. Primary immunodeficiency diseases in adults. *Journal of the American Medical Association*, Jan 7, 1998; 179 (1): 58-61.

25. Lederman, H. M. The clinical presentations of primary immunodeficiency diseases. *Clinical Focus on Primary Immune Deficiencies*, 2000, 2 (1): 2.

26. Cone, M. Bear Trouble. *Smithsonian*, April 2003: 68-74.

27. Leblond, V. S., Hontela, A. Effects of in vitro exposures to cadmium, mercury, zinc, and 1-(2-chlorophenyl)-1-(4-chlorophenyl)-2,2-dichloroethane on steroidogenesis by dispersed interrenal cells of rainbow trout (Oncorhynchus mykiss). *Toxicology and Applied Pharmacology*, 1999; 157(1):16-22

28. Norris, D. O., Donahue, S., Dores, R. M., et al. Impaired adrenocortical response to stress by brown trout, Salmo trutta, living in metal-contaminated waters of the Eagle River, Colorado. *General and Comparative Endocrinology*, 1999; 113 (1):1-8

29. Cancer Facts, National Cancer Institute: http:cis.nci.nih.gov/fact/3_17.htm

30. Gruber, C. J., Tschugguel, W., Schneeberger, C., Huber, J.C. Production and actions of estrogens. *New England Journal of Medicine*, 2002; 346 (5): 340-352.

31. Gunin, A. G., Sharov A. A. Proliferation, mitosis orientation, and morphogenetic changes in the uterus of mice following chronic treatment with both estrogen and glucocorticoid hormones. *The Journal of Endocrinology*, 2001; 169: 23-31.

Protocol

MALE:

A: BLOOD
Cortisol
T3
T4
Total Estrogen
IgA, IgM, IgG

B: URINE
24-hour urine collection (check for active hormones

C: BASAL METABOLIC TEMPERATURE
Upon waking, place thermometer in axilia for 10 minutes before getting up. Normal temperature should be 97.8 -98.2 degrees.

D: BLOOD, URINE & HAIR ANALYSIS FOR HEAVY METALS AND TOXINS

FEMALE:

A: BLOOD
Cortisol
T3
T4
Total Estrogen
IgA, IgM, IgG

B: URINE
24-hour urine collection (check for active hormones)

C: BASAL METABOLIC TEMPERATURE
Upon waking, place thermometer in axilia for 10 minutes before getting up. Normal temperature should be 97.8 - 98.2 degrees. This is only accurate in menstruating women from second to fourth day.

D: BLOOD, URINE & HAIR ANALYSIS FOR HEAVY METALS AND TOXINS

IMPORTANT CONSIDERATIONS

Determining the source or sources of body estrogen is critical. While the ovaries do indeed produce estrogen, they are far from the only source. Non-ovarian estrogen may enter the body or be produced in any of the following ways:

- The adrenal cortex (zona reticularis and possible interface layer) both produce forms of estrogen.
- Ingesting soy protein may raise estrogen levels, since soy contains estradiol. The amount of soy ingested seems to make no difference; any soy protein may be enough to push a estrogen prominent person into estrogen dominance.
- The enzyme aromatase converts DHEA, DHEAS and various androgens to estrogen in the tissue.

CAUTIONS

- Taking calcium supplements can bind thyroid hormone if the two enter the body simultaneously. Even though lab results indicate normal levels of thyroid in the blood, the patient's system may still be thyroid deprived if the hormone is bound by calcium. If both supplements are necessary they should be taken six to eight hours apart.
- Aspirin and other medications containing salicylates may cause severe gastritis in patients undergoing steroid therapy.
- Any patient undergoing steroid therapy should be monitored regularly for fructosamine to determine if an early onset or acceleration of diabetes

mellitis may be occurring. The steroid will not cause diabetes mellitis, but it may accelerate disease onset.

- **Patients should monitor their blood pressure morning, noon, and night, since thyroid therapy may raise blood pressure levels.** Patients with an unidentified pre-coronary condition may be at risk. Those patients with an identified cardiac disease should have thyroid medication dosages adjusted accordingly, and contact their physician immediately should tachycardia or arrhythmia occur. (See Therapy Possibilities, pp. 52, 53.)

PATIENTS WHO HAVE BEEN REGULATED SHOULD AVOID THE FOLLOWING:
- **Birth control pills with estrogen**
- **Foods that contain estrogen**
- **Toxins** (if possible)
- **Xenoestrogens** (from black plastic, etc.)
- **Stress.** If stress cannot be avoided and there are changes in estrogen and immunogolubulins during a high stress period extra hydrocortisone may be indicated to address the adrenaline production, which uses hydrocortisone as a catalyst.

MEASURE PRIMARY E-I LEVELS BEFORE MEASURING OTHER HORMONES AND SUBSTANCES

If the Endocrine-Immune panel is run first and the patient's levels for cortisol, total estrogen, IgA, IgG, and IgM and thyroid are normalized by appropriate treatment and supplements, the normalized blood levels may provide a more realistic baseline for evaluating other hormones and substances. Attempting to measure them without first normalizing the endocrine-immune blood imbalances may well yield confusing results.

- **The endocrine system regulates the immune system.** Measurements should reflect how hormones in the system are affecting not only the adrenal-pituitary-hypothalamic axis, but how they are regulating the immune system, not just blood hormone levels per se. Even with proper hormone supplementation the availability of the hormone may depend on the patient's ability to absorb through the gut wall.

FACTORS WHICH MAY LIMIT ABSORPTION:
- **Food sensitivities**
- **Digestive enzyme deficiencies,** and
- **Ingesting oil-based supplements** (These can coat the gut and limit or eliminate the availability of digestive hormone).
- **IgA deficiency**

REGULAR TESTING IS NECESSARY
- **Patients should be tested regularly during and after treatment to monitor progress,** particularly if there is risk of a disease like diabetes, which may be accelerated by steroid use. A blood test will reveal whether or not the supplementation or treatment is maintaining the status quo, improving the patient's health, or contributing to ill health.
- **Measuring the E-I blood panel is simple.** Running the tests can do no harm; drawing the blood for the panel is no more invasive than drawing blood for a standard CBC and lood chemistry. Having the E-I's results at one's disposal does not require any particular action. However, I have found those results invaluable in determining the course of treatment that will best help my patients achieve health, comfort, and a long and happy life.

I offer the specifics of the E-I panel and treatment protocol in the hope that it will provide veterinarians and physicins with added information, and promote better health for their patients. I welcome information and suggestions from those interested in exploring this treatment plan more fully. I urge members of the general public who feel they or their animals may benefit from this treatment plan to contact a qualified physician or veterinarian and discuss the possibilities it may offer.

Blood Tests and Evaluations

TESTING FOR NON-OVARIAN ESTROGEN

An accurate reading for non-ovarian estrogen in women can be obtained by measuring estrogen levels twice within the menstrual cycle:

- First on the seventh day of the cycle, when estrogen is lowest,
- Then again on the twenty-first day of the cycle, when estrogen is highest. The degree of variation probably indicates endogenous and exogenous non-ovarian estrogen.

HANDLING THE BLOOD SAMPLES

- Fill the red top serum separator tube and spin the sample down.
- Refrigerate the serum sample immediately, ship it to the lab refrigerated, keep it cold at the lab, and run it while still cool.
- Blood that has warmed to room temperature at any point in the process may yield false high hormone and antibody levels.

The following factors can affect blood hormone and antibody levels, and should be included in evaluating lab results. Keep in mind that:

- **Estrogen levels will be higher if the patient:**
  - Uses birth control pills or hormone supplements
  - Has ingested soy protein and other estrogen-containing foods.
  - Has ingested or been exposed to toxins
  - Is experiencing stress
- **Normally with estrogen dominance and B cell deregulation all antibody levels will be depressed. If one level is depressed and the others normal or high lab error must be considered.**

SUGGESTED VALUES

I would suggest these values as a starting point (see Figs. 1 and 2). Highs and lows will certainly need to be modified based on physicians' clinical experiences and patient results.

FIGURE 1
PROPOSED "NORMAL" RANGES FOR MALES

| TOTAL ESTROGEN | CORTISOL | THYROID | | IMMUNOLOGY | | |
		T3	T4	IgA	IgG	IgM
40-115 PG/ML	5.5-20 UG/DL	86-187 NG/DL	4.5-12 UG/DL	70-320 MG/DL	700-1,500 MG/DL	55-200 MG/DL

FIGURE 2
PROPOSED "NORMAL" RANGES FOR FEMALES

| TOTAL ESTROGEN | | CORTISOL | THYROID | | IMMUNOLOGY | | |
			T3	T4	IgA	IgG	IgM
1-10 DAYS	61-394 PG/ML	5.5-20 UG/DL	86-187 NG/DL	4.5-12 UG/DL	70-320 MG/DL	700-1,500 MG/DL	55-200 MG/DL
11-20 DAYS	122-437 PG/ML						
21-30 DAYS	156-350 PG/ML						
PREPUBERTAL LESS THAN 40 PG/ML							
POSTMENOPAUSAL LESS THAN 40 PG/ML							

Therapy Possibilities for Humans

If identifying the hormonal imbalance is the first step, choosing the appropriate therapy options for each patient is the second. Here is a suggested treatment regimen. The broad treatment outline is very similar for each patient: the hormones must be balanced, which may mean hydrocortisone supplements, thyroid supplements, some combination of the two, or even other hormones if indicated.

While the broad outlines remain much the same for many patients, the actual implementation will need to be shaped by veterinarian and physician decisions guided by patient response to the medications prescribed. I have repeatedly found in my work with animals that patients' systems are highly individual. Physicians using the program report the same thing. Reading the blood tests provides a picture of the problem; listening to the patient's body as it reacts to therapy reveals whether the problem is being addressed effectively. Options exist. If the first medication causes discomfort or uncomfortable side effects, explore those options. The focus of treatment is correcting the imbalance, re-regulating the immune system, and helping each patient's body to work at optimum level.

HYDROCORTISONE REPLACEMENT ALTERNATIVES

Synthetic steroids
- Predisone or Prednisolone
- Medrol
- Triamcinolone

Synethetic steroids typically have a twenty-four action, so need be administered just once a day.

Synthetic hydrocortisone
- Cortef (a synthetic hydrocortisone)

Synthetic hydrocortisone is normally administered three to four times a day, in dosages of 2.5 to 5 mg. If insomnia occurs, the fourth (evening) dose of the day can be omitted.

Natural hydrocortisone

Natural hydrocortisone, which appears to be biologically identical to the hydrocortisone the body naturally produces, is placed in combination with olive oil and is absorbed through the lymphatic system. It tends not to cause steroid hepatopathy. I have used an an ultra extract of soy or yams in my animal practice, and had

excellent results. While products including soy plant materials contribute to estrogen dominance, the ultra extract I use as a hydrocortisone supplement has had all plant material removed.

While blood tests do not reflect synthetic steroids, they do reflect natural hydrocortisone, since it appears to be biologically identical to the body's own hydrocortisone.

Natural hydrocortisone supplements are initially administered three times a day at a beginning level of 5 mg dosage three times a day. If insomnia occurs, give 5 mg twice a day, with the last dose being given no later than 6 o'clock p.m.

WHY THYROID REPLACEMENT?
- The patient may have a deficiency in T3/T4
- T3/T4 may be bound by elevated estrogen levels
- T4 transference into active T3 may not occur if there is a hydrocortisone imbalance

Active and storage thyroid (T3 and T4) supplements generally need to accompany the steroid therapy when it is administered to humans. This ensures that the estrogen dominant lock on the thyroid hormone can be superseded. The thyroid hormone also helps ensure that the hydrocortisone is processed properly within a 24-hour period. If proper thyroid therapy is not utilized the cortisone will go from a physiological level to a pharmacological level and harm the patient.

One grain (or 60 mg) of T3/T4 supplementation is usually sufficient for a 100 pound patient, if there are no absorption issues and no allergies that relate to the source of the thyroid hormone, i.e. porcine or bovine thyroid tissue. Since people, unlike animals, can develop cardiac problems on thyroid hormone it is imperative that each patient treated use a battery operated blood pressure cuff and keep an active daily journal, measuring blood pressure and heart rate morning, noon, and night.

Thyroid therapy may raise blood pressure levels in unidentified pre-coronary patients, which could lead to cardiac difficulties. If cardiac issues are present or suspected it is safer to begin T3/T4 dosages at 15 to 30 mg per day. The level can be increased by 15 mg (one quarter grain) every ten days, if necessary. Regulation may proceed more slowly, but the patient will be safer.

Patients should also be informed that excess T3/T4 dosages may cause arrhymthia and tachycardia. If this occurs they should notify their physician immediately, and a blood test should be done immediately. In this case waiting the normal two-three week waiting period before evaluation is unacceptable.

With catastrophic diseases that definitely need hydrocortisone and T3/T4 supplementation an aromatase inhibitor should be considered. Other hormones, like DHEA, DHEAS and androgenic hormones may be converted to total estrogen by aromatase in the tissue. If a patient's life is in jeopardy there is no reason not to use an aromatase inhibitor to somewhat guarantee that endogenous hormones are not metabolized into additional total estrogen.

EVALUATING THE TREATMENT

The E-I test needs to be repeated 2-3 weeks after the initial evaluation to verify that the patient is absorbing correctly, and that levels are falling within the normal range. From then on, the test should be run every 2 to 3 weeks until the patient is stable, at which the time frequency can be reduced to every six months.

TROUBLESHOOTING

Indications that the therapy will or will not work should show up by the second blood test at two to three weeks (about a month after therapy has begun). If total estrogen, IgA, IgG and IgM levels remain the same it is likely that the oral medication is not entering the system. In this instance a combination of Triamcinolone and Depomedrol often needs to be injected intramus-

cularly. The T3/T4 hormones continue by mouth. Immunoglobulin levels should be checked again in two to three weeks.

Once the IgA level reaches 70 mg/dl or higher the patient can be switched from injectible steroids to oral steroids, at which time it will take five to seven days to reach a regulatory level.

Three weeks after beginning the oral cortisone total estrogen, IgA, IgG and IgM levels need to be measured again. If the levels have not changed, the oral hydrocortisone is likely not being absorbed, and further injections are indicated. T3/T4 dosages should be increased to the point where monthly injections will normalize the system.

If the total estrogen and immunoglobulins are better but not perfect the hydrocortisone level should be increased 2.5 to 5 mg over the current dosage two to three times a day. Three weeks later blood estrogen and immunoglobulin levels should to be checked again, and the dosage further adjusted up or down if necessary. At this point in time if the patient is feeling well and the medical disorder is in remission levels need to be continued as is.

About the Author

Alfred J. Plechner, D.V.M., a 1966 graduate of the University of California-Davis School of Veterinary Medicine, has practiced in West Los Angeles for nearly forty years. California Animal Hospital, where he has been an owner practitioner for thirty-six years, has been ranked among the top 1 percent of animal clinics in the United States.

Early in his career Dr. Plechner developed a special interest in nutrition, allergy, and the relationship of hormone-immune imbalances to disease in dogs, cats, and horses. His research and clinical findings have been published in veterinary and human medical journals as well as popular animal magazines.

His most recent book, *Pets at Risk: From Allergies to Cancer, Remedies for an Unsuspected Epidemic* (co-author Martin Zucker, Newsage Press 2003), explains extensively his clinical findings and treatment program for correcting imbalances in pets. Carvel Tiekert, D.V.M., founder of the American Holistic Veterinary Medical Association, hails Dr. Plecher's clinical findings and treatment program. "This book presents us with

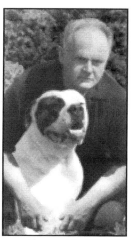

DR. PLECHNER
AND BRUISER

a way of evaluating and treating our animal patients with all kinds of problems related to dysfunctional immune systems. My initial experiences with the protocol have been extremely gratifying."

Dr. Plechner's first book, *Pet Allergies,* was co-authored with Martin Zucker in 1986. The *Seattle Times* described it as "a superb, provocative, wake-up call to American pet owners."

Over the years, Dr. Plechner has formulated a number of widely distributed commercial diets for food-sensitive pets, including the first non-meat and lamb and rice recipes.

Dr. Plechner can be reached through his website: www.drplechner.com.

Made in the USA
Lexington, KY
24 February 2018